MEDICAL MEDDLERS, MEDIUMS AND MAGICIANS

MEDICAL MEDDLERS, MEDIUMS AND MAGICIANS

THE VICTORIAN AGE OF CREDULITY

DR KEITH SOUTER

ILLUSTRATED BY LAURA MATINE

For Jon, my son-in-law
&
In memory of my great grandfather, who for a time
actually was a Victorian music hall performer.
Keith Souter

For my lovely boy, Kester.
Laura Matine

First published 2012

The History Press
The Mill, Brimscombe Port
Stroud, Gloucestershire, GL5 2QG
www.thehistorypress.co.uk

British Library Cataloguing in Publication Data.
A catalogue record for this book is available from the British Library.

ISBN 978 0 7524 6115 1

Typesetting and origination by The History Press
Printed in Great Britain
Manufacturing managed by Jellyfish Print Solutions Ltd

CONTENTS

ACKNOWLEDGEMENTS

Writing a book is never a solitary venture. There are always many people working away backstage who help in their different ways to get the show on the road.

The analogy of a show is entirely appropriate to this book, considering that many of the people described in this book were performers in one way or another. And so I begin my thanks with the late great David Nixon, whose television magic shows sparked off my lifelong interest in conjuring.

My agent Isabel Atherton is, I am sure, a conjuror herself, for she seems to produce book deals with the dexterity of a skilled prestidigitator. She worked her magic with this book and for that I give her my thanks.

Simon Hamlet was the senior commissioning editor at The History Press who accepted the book proposal and started the process of putting the show on stage. He was succeeded by Abbie Wood and then by Lindsey Smith, all of whom have been most helpful in refining the work and preparing it for its dress rehearsal. Mark Beynon, my editor, completed the grooming and helped prepare the book for its public appearance. I am grateful to them all.

A huge vote of thanks to the talented Laura Matine, who has so skilfully illustrated the book and captured the Victorian atmosphere so successfully. It has been a pleasure to work with her once again.

And finally, thanks as ever to my wife Rachel, who makes everything worthwhile.

AUTHOR'S NOTE

In deciding to write a book about the Victorian Age of Credulity I should explain that I have no intention of disparaging the people who lived during the reign of Queen Victoria. Indeed, I confess to being a huge admirer of the Victorian age.

When I was a youngster I devoured the works of Charles Dickens and Sir Arthur Conan Doyle. Dickens painted the picture of the Victorian era up until his death in 1870, then Conan Doyle gave us Sherlock Holmes and the colourful world of the London underworld. While as a teenager I wanted to follow in the footsteps of the great detective, it was actually to be the path of his friend and confidant Dr John H. Watson that I followed as an adult, when I entered medical school to begin a career in medicine.

Yet I also had a fascination for all things to do with conjuring. As a 7-year-old such was my passion for the magic art that I joined the David Nixon Magic Club and proudly carried the membership card and wore the badge to show everyone. In the 1950s and '60s David Nixon was *the* magician and I imagined that one day perhaps I would emulate him by performing feats of magic.

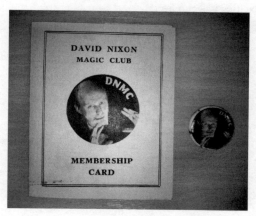

The David Nixon Magic Club membership card and badge.

Having always had a strong sense of history I have researched the history of science and medicine and the history of magic for many years. I studied about the sleep temples of ancient Greece, the Roman hospitals, the anatomy teaching schools of Georgian England. I read about the great magicians of the past; I studied their books, their shows and strove to learn their secrets. Yet between these two areas of study I found myself becoming fascinated by the Victorians' approach to death and their interest in the occult and spiritualism.

As I immersed myself in a study of the Victorian age it became increasingly clear that people at that time were incredibly open to new ideas and were often extremely credulous. This credulity extended across all areas of life, but especially so in the areas of medicine, belief and entertainment. There were practitioners who were willing to prey on people's gullibility. These were the *Medical Meddlers, Mediums and Magicians* of the *Victorian Age of Credulity*.

While there may not seem to be an immediate link between these three groups, on closer inspection there is. You could say that within all three groups there were people who deliberately set out to deceive and to profit from their deception. Magicians, as entertainers, were honest about their deception. They were illusionists, actors playing the part of magicians and wizards. Out and out quacks and fraudulent mediums were anything but honest, for they preyed on people's weaknesses. As we shall see in this book, there were overlaps of all three groups in many instances.

In my opinion, the magicians come out of this little study with the greatest dignity, for as professional deceivers themselves they were often responsible for unmasking and exposing those who claimed to have powers that they did not. In an age of credulity they used their skills to educate and to discredit dishonest swindlers.

This book is the fruit of those studies, which has been simmering along in the back of my mind for far too long. So welcome, I hope that you enjoy the journey back into the days of Victorian yesteryear when the world was a more mysterious and intensely exciting place to live.

Keith Souter

INTRODUCTION

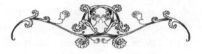

Before We Lift The Curtain Or Attempt To Part The Misty Veil
An introduction to credulity

Before we start on our journey it would make sense to consider some of the reasons why the Victorians were so willing to believe in the claims of quacks and the table knocking that they heard during séances, and be convinced that the illusionists who performed in the theatres and music halls were capable of actual magic.

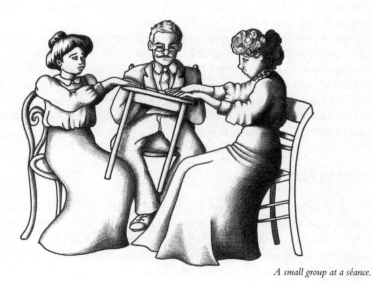

A small group at a séance.

During the Victorian age the thirst for knowledge and discovery seemed insatiable. Built upon the Industrial Revolution and the Age of Enlightenment it was a great age ruled over by Queen Victoria and, until his death, her husband Albert, the prince consort. In all areas of life pioneers were pushing back the frontiers of knowledge and improving transport, communication, engineering and architecture. Steam power, gas, electricity, anaesthetics and aseptic surgery promised to make the world a better and safer place to live in. Perhaps most significantly, Charles Darwin developed his theory of evolution and published his ground-breaking book *On the Origin of Species*, which shook the very foundations of religion and belief.

The expanding British Empire meant that maps were continually being redrawn in order to show the spread of pink, showing the extent of the empire upon which the sun never set. People were proud and patriotic. Yet it was also a time when children were sent up chimneys, down mines and made to work unbearably long hours when they should have been playing or learning. It was a time when we had workhouses, appalling slums and prisons where both men and women were sent to do hard labour. This huge inequality in society stimulated men and women to do their utmost to bring about social reforms. It was a slow process.

It is perhaps because there was so much change going on and so many discoveries being made that people were open to all sorts of ideas. The truth is that although advances were being made in many sciences, medicine lagged behind. The germ theory of disease was not proposed until late in the nineteenth century, so there was fertile ground for all manner of theories about health. Medicine was a very inexact science and until 1858 the medical profession was totally unregulated.

Medical meddlers or out and out quacks peddled all manner of potions, nostrums and elixirs to cure all sorts of ailments, from baldness to impotence, from piles to gangrene, and from syphilis to death itself.

Death was of course always on people's minds, since there was incredibly high infant mortality, there were epidemics and there were casualties from the many wars that were fought to extend and protect the empire's dominions. Mediums and clairvoyants preyed on the recently bereaved in séance parlours and village halls and seemed adept at parting the misty veil between the world of the living and the dead. They talked with the departed and produced ghostly phenomena or even manifested the spirits themselves.

CREDULITY

Not all of the people who practiced outré medical arts were quacks and charlatans. Neither were all of the mediums deliberate frauds. Certainly the vast majority of conjurors and illusionists never claimed to be anything other than entertainers, yet there are common threads linking the three areas. The backdrop against which they were all played was that of human credulity.

Credulity means the willingness to believe in something or in someone based on fairly scant evidence. While it can be considered as a good quality, more often people regard it as a weakness. Children naturally tend to be trusting in their parents and their family, but they have to be taught to be wary of strangers. This is sensible, since not everyone is trustworthy. Adults who remain credulous could be vulnerable to others who may gain some advantage by wilfully deceiving them.

People do vary in their credulity. It is a complex matter that has many elements. Although it is an artificial gradation you can virtually divide people into four types – sceptical, open-minded, willing dupe, or totally gullible. I am sure that you will recognise friends and family who fall into one or other group.

Credulity can also vary in any individual from time to time. Belief in a god is an example. When people are bereaved they are more likely to seek solace in religion, in the belief that the deceased will not simply cease to exist. Similarly, faced with illness that will not respond to medication they may accept the assurance about some other treatment from someone who seems knowledgeable, or from someone who received benefit from that treatment.

A gambler may be an out and out rationalist, yet when having a flutter he may ask Lady Luck to help him. People believe in lucky charms, talismans and good-luck tokens.

In the Victorian age we knew less about the laws of science or about the causes of illness. People may have felt less secure about reaching their allotted life span, and they were less sure that illnesses were not under the control of deities or spirits. The world was an altogether more mysterious place and many more things were possible.

PLAUSIBILITY

This goes hand in hand with credulity. Plausibility means whether something seems to be possible or acceptable.

When someone tries to persuade you to use a particular treatment then the way they explain its benefits will be extremely important. If they can persuade you that it sounds plausible then there is a good chance that it will work.

If someone gives a good explanation of the way in which the living and the dead can both exist then you may be persuaded to attend a séance. You may be willing to accept all that you see and hear at the event.

A medical theory or a philosophy, if it seems in accord with known science and the currently accepted understanding of the way that things work, will seem more plausible. This was the case with phrenology, the study of character through analysis of the contours of the lumps and bumps on the skull. It seemed plausible based on the Victorian understanding about the brain and the huge interest in anthropology that was generated by explorers and those who followed Darwin's theories about evolution. Similarly, homoeopathy, the system of medicine based upon the principle of treating 'like with like', seemed intensely credible. Interestingly, of the two practices, phrenology (which seemed most plausible) died out while homoeopathy still thrives around the world, albeit continually dogged by controversy.

SUGGESTIBILITY

This is an interesting phenomenon that links credulity with plausibility. In normal consciousness we use various mental mechanisms that together make up our critical faculty. We use this in order to balance our credulity with what seems to be plausible.

In a hypnotic trance, one goes into a relaxed state in which the critical faculty ceases to operate at a normal level. For example, if you are given a pencil to hold when you are fully conscious, and told that the pencil will gradually get hotter and hotter, then your critical faculty will tell you that this is not plausible because pencils have no means of getting hotter of their own accord. If you are then put into a light hypnotic trance and again handed the pencil with the same suggestion that it will get hotter and hotter, then you probably would feel it getting hotter and hotter until you could no longer hold it. The pencil has not become hot, of course, rather your critical faculty has ceased to work so that you do not criticise the suggestion and it seems to be plausible. The result is that you respond to the suggestion.

This is not to say that during Victorian times people were hypnotised into thinking that things would work. There are other circumstances in which suggestibility increases. One such condition is in crowds united for a single purpose. An audience will often accept the illusion of the magician. A group listening to someone expound about the merits of a patent treatment at a medicine show may respond to the suggestions given. Similarly, people attending a séance may enter a trance-like state and suspend their critical faculty, so that they become open to all manner of things that they see and hear.

THE PLACEBO EFFECT

This is highly relevant to our consideration about medical meddlers. A placebo is an ineffective drug or treatment that somehow makes the patient feel better. The world comes from the Latin *placere*, meaning 'to please'.

The placebo effect is a fascinating phenomenon, possibly the most fascinating phenomenon in medicine. For some reason (possibly for many reasons, including those that we have just considered) an individual will respond to an inactive agent in a very positive manner. Nowadays placebos are used in scientific trials, usually double-blind trials, in which neither the patient nor the doctor knows whether they are being given an active agent or a placebo. This sort of trial is used to assess whether a drug (the active agent) is superior to the placebo, i.e., better than nothing. The problem is that a placebo response can occur in anything between 25 and 70 per cent of cases. The frequently reported placebo response is 30 per cent, but it depends upon many factors. In general, the more dramatic the treatment, the greater the placebo response. It is also thought that the more the treatment is 'sold' by the enthusiasm of the practitioner the greater the placebo effect will be.

ILLUSION

Magicians specialise in the art of illusion. Essentially they present an effect that seems to operate by unseen means, by the power of magic. It is, however, just a trick. The point is that the observer sees the effect and draws his or her own conclusion. For example, a woman may be sawn in half. The audience sees it happen, yet everyone knows that it cannot possibly have occurred without fatal consequences to the magician's assistant. The mind therefore interprets it as either a feat of magic, or of a skilful illusion.

We lay a great deal of importance upon what we see. In the context of a magic show you would accept the illusion as a magic trick. In the context of a medicine show it could be a very different conclusion. If you see someone hobble on stage on crutches and receive some treatment, be that a swig of elixir, a massage or some other treatment, before standing up straight and throwing away the crutches, then you could be forgiven for accepting what you saw as reality rather than a trick.

In the darkened room of a séance a ghostly manifestation would seem to be more real than a similar manifestation on a magician's stage.

The context of the illusion and the manner in which it is presented will have a different impact upon individuals. The showmen, medical meddlers and mediums of the Victorian age had an awareness of this.

HOW LEGENDS SPREAD

Word of mouth has a very powerful effect on people. Once something or someone gains a reputation it can spread like wildfire. This was certainly the case with many of the medical meddlers who gained fame (or infamy) and fortune in days gone by. News about Dr Elisha Perkins and his tractors literally crossed the Atlantic and made him a fortune. Dr Ward's drops similarly made him a rich man. People flocked to hear Mrs Maria Hayden, the American medium, when she came to London in 1852.

The most famous magic illusion is the 'Indian Rope Trick'. In his book *The Rise of the Indian Rope Trick*, Peter Lamont tracks down the origin of the legendary illusion and explains how it grew in the telling.

All successful medical meddlers, mediums and magicians have to be aware of the importance of self-publicity if they want to become legends.

SELF-DELUSION

In psychiatry a delusion is defined as a false, fixed belief that is impervious to reason. It is not a normal state. It usually occurs as part of an underlying mental condition. A self-delusion is not necessarily a symptom of a mental condition. It can quite simply be a state whereby someone comes to believe in a system or theory that they practice. They come to believe that their system or theory is correct and that any effect anyone derives from its application is due to their ability to use the system, or is a validation of the system itself.

That is to say that someone could practice a type of medicine using a set of gadgets like the tractor rods that had been made by a supposed expert, such as Dr Elisha Perkins (who we shall consider in Chapter 2 The Golden Age of Quackery), and attribute results to the tractors, and not to the other factors that we have looked at in this introduction.

I do believe that this was the case with some of the practitioners of the various methods or philosophies that we will meet in the book. While some were utter rogues, others were credulous dupes. Essentially, there are likely to have been two types of practitioner (of both quack medicine and mediumship): those who knowingly deceived and those who were self-deluded as to the reason why they enjoyed their success.

AND FINALLY

I must clarify, however, that as to the question of whether or not the spirit does survive death I make no pronouncement either way. Nor do I have any view on modern-day spiritualism. I am sure that today, just as during the Victorian era, there are many people who are totally convinced that this is a reality and that contact with spirits is quite genuine. My only concern is with the fraudulent practices that unscrupulous mediums used during the Victorian age to dupe people who desperately wanted to believe.

And so now, let the curtain rise and the show and the séance begin!

PART ONE

MEDICAL
MEDDLERS

1

A MAJESTIC MEDICAL MEDDLER

In consideration whereof, and for the ease, Comfort, Succour, Help, Relief, and Health of the King's poor Subjects, Inhabitants of this Realm, now pained or diseased: … It shall be lawfull to every person being the King's subject, having knowledge and experience of the nature of Herbs, Roots and Waters, or of the operation of same …, to practice, use and minister in and to any outward sore, uncome, wound, apostemations, outward swelling or disease, any herb or herbs, oyntments, baths, pultes and amplaisters, according to their cunning, experience and knowledge in any of the diseases.

Herbalist's Charter
King Henry VIII, 1542

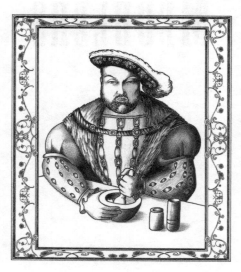

King Henry VIII
was fascinated
by potions.

Throughout the history of medicine the majority of doctors have based their practice upon the accepted knowledge of the day. Those who do not subscribe to this approach but use unorthodox methods inevitably face being ridiculed by their peers or disparaged as *quacks*. The word 'quack' actually comes from 'quacksalver', derived from the Dutch *kwakzalver*. Originally it was used to describe a peddler in ready-made remedies, but eventually it became used as a blanket derogatory term for anyone who made extravagant claims about their expertise or their treatments.

Another derogatory term that was applied was 'mountebank'. The origin of this was from the idea that unlicensed peddlers of medicine and nostrums would mount a bench or small stage at fairs or markets in order to extol about their remedies or their skill.

Of course, no one would ever have proudly claimed themselves to be a quack. Over the years, however, within the ranks of those who have been proclaimed quacks there are to be found many eminent people who did good work and whose inclusion was the result of professional jealousy. Such is the case of the great Dr Ignac Semmelweis (1818–65), a Hungarian physician who saved thousands of women from puerperal fever, an almost always fatal condition in the early nineteenth century, when he advocated that all doctors should wash their hands between conducting post-mortem examinations and visiting the midwifery suites. The orthodox profession was outraged at his audacity and he was effectively forced to leave Vienna.

Equally, there are many who attained fame and fortune in the sure knowledge that they were professing information they did not possess, and who offered treatments that they knew to be well-nigh useless.

But before we delve into the murky waters of medical meddling and the world of quack medicine, we need to look a little at the way that medicine has evolved.

HIPPOCRATES – THE FATHER OF MEDICINE

Hippocrates of Cos (460–377 BC) was a priest physician of the cult of Aesculepius. He was the first doctor to attempt to put medicine on a theoretical basis rather than attributing illness to demonic possession or the displeasure of the gods. He formulated the Hippocratic oath and wrote a body of work that is known as the *Corpus Hippocratum*.

THE HUMORAL THEORY

Hippocrates taught the Doctrine of Humors. This became the dominant theory in medicine until the Renaissance. Essentially, it was believed that there were four fundamental humors or body fluids which determined the state of health of the individual.

These humors were blood, yellow bile, black bile and phlegm. Aristotle had taught that the humors were associated with the four elements of air, fire, earth and water, which in turn were associated to paired qualities of hot, cold, dry and moist. Thus, earth would be dry and cold, water would be wet and cold, fire would be hot and dry, and air would be wet and hot.

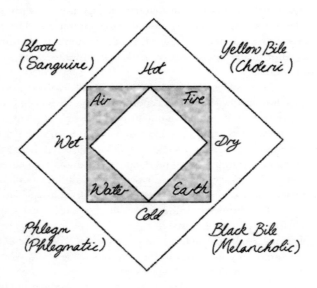

The Doctrine of Humors.

GALEN OF PERGAMMON

Claudius Galenus (AD 131–201), known to history as Galen, was a Greek physician who practiced as a physician to a gladiatorial school and was later personal doctor to the emperor Marcus Aurelius. He developed the Doctrine of Humors further and taught that a proper balance of them was necessary for health. An excess of any humor could be treated by reducing a quality, or by reducing a humor, e.g. bleeding the patient or giving enemas, or treating with various Galenical drugs. An example of a Galenical would contain cucumber, which has cooling properties, because it naturally contains salicylates.

The individual's temperament could also be discerned according to their balance of humors. Thus, sanguine individuals were perceived to have excess blood, choleric individuals had excess yellow bile, melancholics had too much black bile and phlegmatics had excess phlegm. As a philosophical system it had much to commend it and seemed perfectly plausible.

RENAISSANCE MEDICINE

This period saw a spate of scientific discoveries which would gradually discredit the humoral theory. The study of anatomy had been carried out erratically over the centuries, mainly because dissection was considered by the Church to be a desecration and an abomination. Nevertheless, in 1543 Andreus Vesalius of Florence published the world's first anatomically correct treatise on anatomy. This set off a serious study of the body that culminated in William Harvey's discovery of the circulation of the blood in 1616. Doctors began to realise that blood circulated, but there was no equivalent circulation for the other supposed humors.

Then in 1625, Santorio Santorio, a friend of Galileo, invented the thermometer. This really proved to be the nail in the coffin of the humoral theory since for the first time it could be demonstrated that people with hot or cold constitutions in fact both had the same temperature.

One would have thought that the Doctrine of Humors would just disappear at that point. This was not to be, since its *simplicity* and *plausibility* could be put to great use by the medical meddlers during the age of quackery that would follow.

Now let us backtrack a little to the days of the Tudors to consider one of the greatest medical meddlers.

KING HENRY VIII AND THE QUACK'S CHARTER

Medicine in Tudor England was a hotchpotch of medical practice. In 1518 King Henry VIII (1491–1547) conferred a royal charter to found the College of Physicians in London. This was the first attempt to regulate medical practice, albeit only loosely. The College of Physicians was permitted to license physicians to practice.

In 1540 he gave another royal charter to form the Company of Barber-Surgeons, which would eventually become the Royal College of Surgeons in 1800. Its function was to license surgeons.

By granting these two charters, King Henry VIII had effectively given the physicians and the surgeons the social status and recognition that they had sought. The physicians thought themselves to be socially superior to the surgeons, who in turn thought themselves to be superior to the apothecaries and other people who plied a trade. An effect of these charters, however, was that it was seen to give the physicians and the surgeons a monopoly on the preparation of medicines. Poor people could not afford the expensive preparations containing precious metals and minerals that the physicians and surgeons prescribed. Interestingly, Henry had some sympathy for them, for he himself was a medical meddler.

In 1542 he granted the Herbalist's Charter, which allowed herbalists, or anyone with knowledge to do so, the right to prepare herbal remedies. Since this effectively gave anyone the right to practice medicine without any interference from the physicians or surgeons, it was derided by the medical profession as being the Quack's Charter.

Undoubtedly, Henry's interest in herbal preparations derived from self-interest. He suffered from leg ulceration for many years. Whether it was a varicose ulcer or a syphilitic ulcer has been debated by historians for many years. Whichever it was, he clearly tried to treat it himself. Indeed, he is known to have been experienced in compounding ointments and making plasters.

He actually collaborated with several doctors and wrote a book on the subject, containing 130 prescriptions. Many of them actually acknowledge that they were 'devised by the King's Majesty'. One prescription for a plaster 'Resolved Humor If There Is Swellgnje In the Legges'.

Another was devised 'for the King's Grace to coole and dry and comfort the member'. It is likely that this and other similar ones were created by him to soothe and salve the king's own intimate person, his sexual life being an important part of his very being.

King Henry VIII had set the scene with this charter. The real medical meddling was soon to start.

2

THE GOLDEN AGE OF QUACKERY

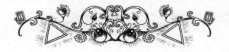

Before you take his drops or pills,
Take leave of friends and make your will.

Satirical caution about Joshua Ward's 'Pill and Drop', 1760

The Restoration of King Charles II in 1660 could be said to mark the beginning of the Golden Age of Quackery. It was a period that lasted for over a century and a half and quite naturally merged into what I describe as the Victorian Age of Credulity.

After the puritanical rule of the Commonwealth between 1647 and 1660, during which time even Christmas celebrations had been banned, there was a general relaxing of social strictures. Many doctors started actively seeking patients and building their practices. They were not alone, however, for this was England where it was perfectly legal after King Henry VIII Herbalist's Charter to practice medicine under Common Law. Accordingly, they found themselves in competition with many unqualified practitioners, many of whom came to England from abroad, claiming that they had been granted royal patronage by King Charles while he had been in exile.

KING CHARLES II AND DR GODDARD'S DROPS

One respected physician by the name of Dr Jonathan Goddard (1617–75), one of the first fellows of King Charles II's recently created Royal Society in 1660, was not a quack, but he did profit most handsomely from some shrewd business practice with the king, which today would be regarded as highly unethical.

Dr Goddard had been a Member of Parliament, an army surgeon during the Civil War and personal physician to Oliver Cromwell. He was to become a Professor of Physick at Gresham College. He had invented a secret elixir which he marketed as 'Goddard's Drops', advocating their use for virtually everything. King Charles II was clearly impressed with them, for the Treasury warrant book for 16 March 1698 records a payment of £60 'to Peter Hume Esq. without account for the purchase of a quantity of Doctor Goddard's Drops which by the King's commands are to be sent as a present from his Majesty to the Queen of Sweden'.

His majesty was indeed so impressed that he paid Dr Goddard the sum of £6,000 for the secret formula for his wonderful drops. As it turned out the drops were little more than *sal volatile* – simple smelling salts.

QUEEN ANNE AND HER OCULIST

The last Stuart ruler to be crowned was Queen Anne (1665–1714). Coming to the throne at the age of 18, she was not a well woman. Indeed, she actually had to be carried to her coronation because she was suffering from gout. In addition to this she had poor vision all of her life and was often treated by her favourite oculist, one William Read, who in fact was an unmitigated medical meddler or mountebank.

Read was born in Aberdeen and started his working life as a tailor. He was apparently uneducated and barely able to read or write. Despite this, however, he practiced throughout the north of England as an itinerant oculist or eye specialist. Gaining some reputation and some success with his potions and eye washes he moved to London where he set up a practice in the Strand.

One of his handbills proclaimed that he had twenty-one years of experience and that he could treat glaucoma, a condition caused by increased pressure in the eye, could couche cataracts and deal with all manner of suffusions.

History tells us that Queen Anne was extremely impressed by his ministrations and in 1706 knighted him for his services that he had astutely given free to soldiers and seamen.

In that same year he published a book entitled *A Short but Exact Account of all the Diseases Incident to the Eyes With Causes, Symptoms, and Cures, also Practical Observations upon some Extraordinary Diseases of the Eyes*. There were two editions of the book published. Some of it was actually quite accurate, which is not surprising considering that it was all copied from a book published in 1622 by Richard Bannister, a surgeon and oculist of London!

A section about anatomy and physiology were no more than copies of ancient texts. All in all, the book clearly had not been written by anyone with any knowledge of the anatomical discoveries that had been made about the eye by contemporary anatomists. In the main it was a boastful account of his successes with his quack treatment, which he called 'Styptick Water'.

Although he became very successful and very wealthy, his secret eventually came out and he was lampooned in the pamphlets of the day:

Her majesty sure was in a surprise
Or else was very shortsighted
When a tinker was sworn to look after her eyes
And the Mountebank Read was knighted …

When he died in 1715, his wife, Lady Read, continued his work with his Styptick Water. Queen Anne's heir, the Hanoverian King George I, consulted her, but was not impressed with her skills. He gave her a pension and immediately appointed another oculist, Robert Grant. Like Read, he had started life in quite a different trade. He had been a cobbler and somewhere along the way he lost an eye. Perhaps that stimulated him to proclaim himself an eye specialist, for he had no medical qualification whatsoever.

JOANNA STEPHENS AND HER MEDICINE FOR THE STONES

One of the great health problems which caused excruciating pain in past centuries was the agony of bladder stones. Poor diet and dehydration from avoiding the drinking of water and taking wine, beer or porter instead would have made stone formation in the urinary tract a definite possibility. The treatment involved 'cutting for stone', a procedure that filled patients with horror, yet which filled the pockets of the workaday surgeon. Then, in 1735, along came Joanna Stephens and her secret cure for stones.

Joanna Stephens was the daughter of a Berkshire gentleman. In about 1720 she compounded a remedy made from baked eggshells with a decoction of soap and other secret ingredients, with the specific purpose of dissolving kidney and bladder stones. Not surprisingly, people were willing to try anything that would keep them away from the surgeon's knife. Her results were reported to be amazing.

Her cause was championed by Dr David Hartley, who was later to become famous as the originator of the Associationist school of psychology. He suffered from recurrent bladder stones and experimented with the treatment. He wrote a series of papers explaining why eggs were used (since the shells were made of calcium carbonate, which when heated would produce lime, which had been used for the treatment of stones since the days of the Roman writer Pliny) and why soap was needed (because the lime constipated and the soap would counter this). He sincerely believed that Joanna's secret cure would be of incredible benefit to the public. This cry was taken up by the Hon. Edward Carteret, the Postmaster General. Soon other dignitaries attested to its value and Joanna was asked to reveal her secret which was obviously of 'great importance to mankind'. She agreed to do so, for the price of a mere £5,000.

A public subscription was started, which fell short of her fee, but she held firm. Parliament was petitioned and duly agreed to pay her. As agreed, she handed over her secret recipe, which was duly printed in the *London Gazette*. The ingredients consisted of bird and snail shells, carrot seeds, soap, honey and various traditional herbs.

Joanna took the money and lived comfortably and quietly ever after. Her wonder remedy gradually fell from favour, its magic having disappeared when the contents were no longer secret.

MESMER AND ANIMAL MAGNETISM

One of the most charismatic and dramatic figures to grace the annals of medical history was Dr Franz Anton Mesmer (1734–1815). He went to university in Vienna to study divinity, philosophy and law, but changed course and took up the study of medicine. In 1766 he graduated, his doctoral thesis being entitled *De influxu planetarum in corpus humanum – The Influence of the Planets upon the Human Body*.

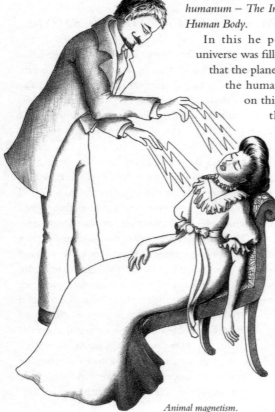

In this he postulated that the whole universe was filled with a magnetic fluid and that the planets exerted an influence upon the human body through their effect on this invisible fluid. He believed that this energy could be harnessed by gifted individuals like himself to correct imbalances in patients. He called this phenomenon 'animal magnetism'.

It was the start of an amazing, if highly controversial, career in medicine that many of his peers considered to be the ultimate in quackery.

Mesmer opened consulting rooms in Vienna and soon built up a lucrative practice that attracted some of the crowned heads of Europe, the nobility and many of the most

Animal magnetism.

influential people of society. At first he believed that this animal magnetism had to be channelled through metal rods, like magnets, in order to influence people. Then, as more people sought his aid, he manufactured a huge drum made of oak filled with water and iron filings, which he called his 'baquet'. Metal rods and wires protruded from the drum and were held by patients against the parts of the body that ailed them. Magnetised metal plates could also be held or placed over painful or paralysed parts. Mesmer would then enter the room, which hummed with violin music, stare into the patients eyes and make passes over their bodies with a metal rod that he carried like a wand, or touch them with it.

The results were nothing short of astonishing. People fainted or seemed to have fits with such frequency that the room was known as the 'hall of convulsions'. Anyone so affected could generally be guaranteed a cure. Often they would be carried by servants to a side room and ministered to until Mesmer came to give them individual treatment. His patients included Mozart, the Empress Maria Theresa and, most significantly, a blind pianist, Marie Therese Paradis, who had been blind since birth. This last case he cured – much to his cost!

There were two problems. First, when this young girl could see, the seeming magic that surrounded her also disappeared. While people marvelled at her ability to play by touch alone, they were less impressed by her ability now that she could see. In addition, she received state benefits because of her disability, which would be withdrawn if she could see. The result was that her parents demanded that Mesmer should stop treating her. When he did so, she of course relapsed.[1] His critics were quick to seize on this, saying that he had merely implanted suggestions into her mind that she could see when she had not seen anything at all. Others claimed that he had seduced her. At any rate, his reputation was badly affected and he moved to Paris in 1778.

In Paris Mesmer realised that all of the accoutrements, like the baquet and the metal rods, were not necessary, so he abandoned them. Now he believed that he himself was acting as a conductor for the animal magnetism and that he could 'mesmerise' patients with the power of his mind alone. There he also gathered critics, presumably through professional jealousy.

So great was the furore that was whipped up against him that in 1784 King Louis XVI established a committee to investigate Mesmer's claims about animal magnetism. This committee consisted of eminent doctors and scientists of the day, including Benjamin Franklin, Dr Guillotin (who was to design the execution machine that was to claim the head of the king himself just five years later), and Antoine Lavoisier, the great chemist. After researching the method, using one of

1. It is highly likely that she was suffering from a condition that we would nowadays diagnose as an hysterical conversion neurosis. This means that she was not consciously pretending to be blind, but her symptoms would have been induced in order to solve an inner unconscious conflict. It was not until the days of Sigmund Freud that modern medicine developed the concept and understanding of a neurosis.

Mesmer's disciples rather than the man himself, they concluded that there was no evidence for rays of animal magnetism and that the whole phenomenon was nonsensical. Again Mesmer moved, this time to London, where he was unable to establish a practice. Disillusioned, he left for Switzerland where he lived in obscurity until his death in 1815.

Although the committee were quite correct, there are no rays of animal magnetism, they had failed to appreciate that the phenomenon of hypnosis, which is what mesmerism is, takes place entirely in the mind of the patient. In later years it would actually become one of the great therapeutic tools of modern psychiatry. Mesmer's own medical meddling had actually done the phenomenon's image the greatest harm.

MRS SALLY MAPP – BONE-SETTER

Broken bones and dislocations in pre-anaesthetic days were recipes for agony, potential for infection and a very real risk of death. All manner of people plied a trade as bone-setters. Farriers, blacksmiths and itinerant body-shapers or bone-setters provided much-needed care if they were skilled and fast. Equally, they could cause much pain and further damage if they were inept.

Mrs Sally Mapp (d. 1737), known as Crazy Sally Mapp, was one such itinerant bone-setter who rose to celebrity thanks to her treatment of Sir Hans Sloane's niece and to her satirisation at the hands of William Hogarth.

Sally Mapp learned her trade from her father, who was also a bone-setter. She was by all accounts a remarkably ugly woman with a squint and prodigiously strong arms. After arguing with her father she left home and set out on her own, acquiring skills on the way and a reputation for being swift and effective at correcting skeletal deformities, setting broken bones and replacing dislocated joints. So great was her success and the demand for her services that the town of Epsom offered her an income of 100 guineas a year to live and practice there.

In the eighteenth century most qualified physicians and surgeons despised these unqualified practitioners. Sir Hans Sloane, the president of the Royal College of Physicians, was more enlightened and was one of her strongest supporters. He had actually sent his niece to her because of a spinal deformity, presumably a scoliosis. Her success and his support clearly enhanced her reputation. Soon people from all over the country were beating a path to her door. With Hogarth's satirisation of her appearance she enjoyed great celebrity. Indeed, on one occasion while riding in her coach along Kent Road she was mistaken for one of King George II's mistresses. One would have thought that being the mistress of a king would bring a certain social kudos, but this was not the case on this occasion. A mob formed and made threatening moves towards her coach. Angrily, she popped her head through the window of the carriage and cried: 'Damn your bloods, don't you know me? I am Mrs Mapp, the bone-setter.'

The cries of derision changed to cheers of adulation and she was permitted to drive on unmolested.

SIR HANS SLOANE (1660–1753)

This great physician was no medical meddler. In addition to being the president of the most prestigious body, the Royal College of Physicians, he was also a collector of all manner of antiquities. Indeed, he donated most of his collection (apart from some fabulous pieces that he kept back and which can be seen in the Sloane Museum on Lincoln's Inn Fields) to the nation, forming the beginning of the collection that became the British Museum. Sloane Square in London is named after him.

He is worthy of consideration in this chapter not only because of his support for Crazy Sally Mapp, but also because he invented a health drink after he returned from a trip to Jamaica. There he had tasted chocolate, but declared that it was quite nauseating. However, when it was mixed with milk, it became quite pleasant and so he promoted it as his 'medicinal chocolate'. The health-giving qualities of the drink may have disappeared over the years, but it is still popular today as good old-fashioned drinking milk chocolate.

WARD'S PILL AND DROP

Joshua Ward (1684–1761) is the epitome of the eighteenth-century medical meddler. He was born in Guisborough, Cleveland, and went into business in London with his brother as a dry-salter. An ambitious man, Joshua stood for parliament in 1717 and was duly elected as an MP for the constituency of Marlborough. Scrutiny of the election results, however, revealed the inconvenient fact that no one had actually voted for him. Furthermore, the mayor's signature on the return proved to be a forgery. Joshua Ward's political career was, therefore, cut short and he was put in the pillory, and then imprisoned. He was also said to have had some Jacobite sympathy following the unsuccessful uprising of 1715. Understandably, upon his release from prison he fled the country until he received a pardon from King George II.

During his time abroad he claimed to have studied medicine and become a doctor. He also invented a patent medicine that would cure all ills, which he produced as 'Ward's Pill and Drop'. In 1734 he returned to London and set up a lucrative practice while he vigorously started to sell and promote his patent medicine.

In 1736 he had a major breakthrough when several eminent medical men, including himself, were invited to attend upon King George II, who was complaining of a painful swollen right thumb. The physicians and surgeons misdiagnosed his case as gout, but Ward manipulated a dislocated thumb and gained royal thanks and royal patronage. As a result, his medications were granted freedom from the legislation that entitled the Royal College of Physicians to examine all medicines. Not only that, but he was granted the privilege of being able to drive his coach and six through St James's Park. This was royal patronage indeed.

The boom in communications in the eighteenth century, thanks to the printing industry that was flourishing, allowed Ward's Pill and Drop to become widely known and widely used. The prime minister, Sir Robert Walpole, used his medicines as did Lord Chesterfield and Henry Fielding, the novelist. Undoubtedly, the remedies worked for many people and they certainly induced a perspiration reaction, which was generally taken as being necessary in order to facilitate a cure. Ward claimed that they could cure scurvy, syphilis and even cancer.

Ward became fabulously wealthy and engaged in philanthropic works. He endowed two hospitals for the poor and a Magdalene house for fallen women. He was a bachelor all his days and when he died he left a small fortune, a large part of which he left to his servants. His secret formula revealed that his remedies contained a mix of several toxic compounds, including antimony. This would in fact have had some anti-inflammatory properties, so it would have had some success.

Ward was buried in poet's corner in Westminster Abbey and a statue of him can be seen today in the Victoria and Albert Museum in London.

JAMES GRAHAM AND HIS TEMPLE OF HEALTH

One of the most famous of all medical meddlers was Edinburgh-born Dr James Graham (1745–94), who actually studied medicine before leaving university without completing his degree. This in itself was not uncommon in the eighteenth century. From Edinburgh he moved to Doncaster where he worked for a while as an assistant to an apothecary before marrying and then moving to America. There he practiced in the colonies as an oculist and aurist, treating people's eye and ear problems – it was here where he learned about electricity.

Leaving America before the War of Independence broke out, he returned to Europe, travelling around and developing his ideas on health all the time. Then he returned to England and set up a practice in Bath, where he offered all manner of esoteric treatments using vapours, magnetism (both animal magnetism/ mesmerism and actual magnetism) and electricity. He disapproved of alcohol and believed that many ailments came from wearing woollen clothes. He himself is said to have favoured a suit of white linen.

In 1781, bolstered by prestigious clients such as Georgina, Duchess of Devon, he moved to London and opened up his Temple of Health in the Adelphi Terrace, near to the Strand. There he gave lectures on health, sex and beauty, recruiting 'Goddesses of Health' whose purpose was to look beautiful and healthy in scanty clothing. One of the beauties was the 16-year-old Emma Lyons, who would later marry and become Emma Hamilton, mistress to Admiral Horatio Nelson.

One of the main features of the Temple of Health was his Celestial Bed, which had magnets built into it, a mattress stuffed with herbs and stallion hair, and a tilting axis so that it could be directed at any angle. Graham guaranteed to help any childless couple become pregnant. They could pay to spend the night in it. It was also, of course, available to reinvigorate even the most worn out of rakes.

Since Graham treated sexual problems and aimed to help infertile couples, you may imagine that as the world's first sexologist he was somewhat obsessed with all matters sexual. In fact he was personally a rather sober individual more given to abstinence that sexual participation. He seems to have genuinely cared and tried to help. His celestial bed, although regarded by satirists in cartoons, pamphlets and newspapers as the height of quackery, in fact offered more than anything that the orthodoxy of the day could provide. The tilting nature of the celestial bed may indeed have been beneficial in encouraging scanty seminal fluid specimens in the right direction. And in creating an ambience and an expectation it is likely that many of his clients were successful.

Yet Graham's ideas and his behaviour gradually became more eccentric. He advocated fasting, gave demonstrations on mud baths and even gave lectures in an earth-bed, in which he was buried in soil right up to his neck.

His untimely death at the age of 49 was taken by many of his critics as proof that his ideas about health were no more than quackery and that they were clearly responsible for his own demise.

PERKINS' TRACTORS AND TRACTORATION

Dr Elisha Perkins (1741–99) was a country doctor who was born in Norwich, Connecticut in America. In the 1790s, he advertised a medical invention that he claimed was capable of curing all manner of ailments. He modestly called the invention 'Perkins' Metallic Tractors', and the system of medicine that he introduced as 'tractoration'.

Essentially, the metal tractors were two rods of steel and brass, which he claimed were unusual alloys, each tapered at one end. The blunt ends were held by the practitioner and the pointed ends were stroked on the patient's body,

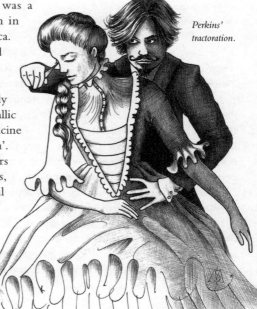

Perkins' tractoration.

down and outwards. It was based on the belief that metal could draw disease out of the body, and Perkins claimed great results with all manner of ailments – toothache, stomach complaints, rheumatism and gout. Gradually he extended the range of conditions to include virtually everything, even paralysis and dropsy. He also claimed that the tractors 'draw off the noxious electrical fluid that lay at the root of suffering'.

Other doctors tried his method and soon tractoration was enjoying a phenomenal success. Grateful patients and other doctors gave glowing testimonials. George Washington, the first president of the United States, tried the method and was apparently an enthusiastic supporter. The Connecticut Medical Society, however, did not concur. They accused him of 'delusive quackery' and judged that he was 'a patentee and user of nostrums'. They accordingly expelled him from their society.

Despite this, other medical societies were supportive and his fortune grew. More than that, his fame spread across the world. When a Danish diplomat returned to Copenhagen he took with him a set of tractors and news of the method. Twelve celebrated surgeons put the method to the test at the Royal Frederick Hospital and reported tractoration a phenomenal success.

His son, Benjamin Perkins, travelled to Britain to spread the word about tractoration. Before long he received the backing of the medical profession and was soon established in a lucrative practice in the West End of London, where smart society sought his services.

In 1798, Benjamin published *The Influence of Metallic Tractors on the Human Body*, and in that same year he placed an advertisement in *The Times* which stated that:

> The tractors, with every necessary direction for using them in Families, may be had for 5 guineas the set, of Mr. Perkins, of Leicester Square; or of Mr. Frederic Smith, Chemist & Druggist, in the Haymarket.

A year later he followed this up with the application of tractoration to animals, when he published a pamphlet *The Family Remedy; or, Perkins's Patent Metallic Tractors, For the Relief of Topical Disease of the Human Body: And of Horses*.

In 1803, Perkins was helped by an aristocratic friend supporter to set up a Perkinsian Institute in Soho for the benefit of the poor, who were not able to shell out the 5 guineas a set. This, however, was not a success. The poor who flocked to the institute for treatment claimed in vast numbers that the tractors did nothing. Perhaps their ailments were more genuine than those of polite society, or perhaps it was because they were not paying for their treatment, but they derided the method. This led some of the medical profession to put it to the test. Some experimented with animals and found tractoration to be valueless.

In 1799 Dr John Haygarth, an eminent physician who had done important work on limiting the spread of smallpox, decided to put the tractors to a scientific test. He compared dummy wooden tractors that were painted to look like metal with a set of 'active' metal tractors. He found that curiously both seemed to get results. His conclusion was that the metal was irrelevant and that there was some other agent at work. This he deduced was none other than the mind. He duly published his findings in a book, *On the Imagination as a Cause & as a Cure of Disorders of the Body*. This is the first recorded demonstration of the placebo effect, even though it had been speculated about as early as 1772.

Tractoration soon declined and Benjamin Perkins retired to his home in America a rich man. Sadly his father, the founder of tractoration, Dr Elisha Perkins, died of yellow fever while on his way to New York to promote a new antiseptic that he had invented to deal with dysentery and sore throats.

Benjamin died in 1810 and the tractors, having no further advocate, fell fully from grace.

Ironically, despite their worthlessness, a set of 'Perkins' Metallic Tractors' will nowadays cost you considerably more than 5 guineas.

THEODOR MYERSBACH THE PISS PROPHET

In medieval medicine the naked-eye examination of a flask of urine had been regarded as one of the main means of diagnosis. 'Uroscopy', as the method was called, was invented by Isaac Judeus (AD 845–940), an Egyptian physician at the School of Medicine at Salerno. A special glass bulbous flask called a 'matula' was developed so that the doctor could look at the urine and check for the presence of blood, discharge or any sediment. He produced a urine colour wheel, a chart on which twenty different colours of urine were represented, each of which would give the doctor a different diagnosis.

This system became one of the dominant features of medicine in the Middle Ages and the matula, the urine flask, became the badge of office of the physician. Indeed, a book published in England in 1541, entitled *The Differences, Causes and Judgements of Urine*, suggested that uroscopy and examination of the pulse were the two most important procedures in medicine.

The advances in science that had been made in the previous century had discredited the method which had fallen into disuse by English physicians, who tended to rely on pulse diagnosis. It was a situation that was quickly seized upon by the medical meddlers.

In the early eighteenth century Theodor Myersbach (1730–98) came to London from Amsterdam and set up as a consulting uroscopist. He claimed to be so successful at diagnosing and treating ailments that he had only to see a specimen of urine to do so. Accordingly, the rich and wealthy were soon despatching their servants with samples to his practice in Berwick Street in Soho, where he would diagnose their problems by swirling their urine in his matula. For an additional fee he would prescribe the appropriate treatments.

He was soon derided by the orthodox profession as a 'piss-prophet' and challenged about his credentials (which were apparently fabricated), his skill and his treatments. One of his most vociferous critics was Dr John Coakley Lettsom, who lambasted Myersbach in a series of pamphlets, that dearly beloved literary medium of the eighteenth century. Myersbach responded in kind and there followed a couple of years of riposte and counter-riposte in the newspapers. The end result was hardly satisfactory for either camp, since the public and the medical profession grew weary of both. Myersbach left England and Lettsom simply made himself unpopular.

A contemporary rhyme summed up the attitude towards the cut and thrust of the pompous physician and the medical meddler:

> When any sick to me apply,
> I physicks, bleeds and sweats 'em;
> If after that they choose to die,
> What's that to me, I Lettsom.

THE COUNT OF CAGLIOSTRO

No account of medical meddling would be complete without some consideration of the greatest mountebank of all, the Count of Cagliostro, who became famous throughout the whole of Europe as a medium, physician and occultist, proclaimed himself to be the discoverer of the Elixir of Youth and the founder of Egyptian Freemasonry. He was fêted by the crowned heads of Europe and conned his way from royal court to royal court. Novels and plays have been written about him by such literary giants as Alexander Dumas, who wrote about him in *Memoirs of a Physician*; Johan Wolfgang von Goethe, who wrote a romance of his life in *Grand Cophta*; and Thomas Carlyle, who gave an account of a celebrated criminal case in *Cagliostro and the Diamond Necklace*. As a charlatan who started as a simple mountebank this colourful character has no equal in the annals of the deceivers.

Count Alessandro Cagliostro (1743–95) was the assumed name of Joseph Balsamo, who was born in Palermo in Sicily, the son of a simple peasant family. Yet despite his humble origin Balsamo was convinced that he had the seeds of greatness in him and he duly set out to make his fortune by whatever means fell open to him. Joseph Balsamo had a knack for spotting openings and, when none were apparent, for making them.

After receiving a rudimentary education that included some instruction in chemistry at a local monastery, he was quick to show off his learning and erudition. He probably also displayed a propensity for dishonesty, for he was expelled from the monastery.

Ever ingenious, however, he developed an aptitude for forgery, which he put to use in the manufacture of counterfeit theatre tickets. This had limited potential, so he turned his hand to forging a will. His most outrageous endeavour in his youth came at the age of 16 when he convinced a local goldsmith, Vincenzo Marano, that he had discovered through the practice of magical arts the whereabouts of a fabulous treasure that was protected by magical creatures. All he asked was a payment of 70 pieces of silver.

One night they went out of the city together to a deserted clearing in a forest where Balsamo drew a circle with some sort of phosphorescent material then cried out a string of mumbo-jumbo, which he assured Marano would protect them. He instructed Marano to dig for the treasure, which the poor fellow did with alacrity. Confederates of the youthful sorcerer then pounced on the goldsmith and beat him close to death. The next morning Marano, fearful that Balsamo had been carried off by the same spirits that had attacked him, called at his home, only to find that he had taken all of his belongings and his silver and had fled the city.

On his travels Balsamo met up with an older man, a Greek alchemist and swindler by the name of Althotas. Together they travelled widely and visited, among other countries, Egypt, Persia and Greece. Balsamo learned much about confidence trickery from the older man, and was by all accounts sad when he passed away when they went to Rhodes. Eventually Balsamo arrived in Malta where, according to his own account (which may of course be taken with a pinch of salt), he studied alchemy under Pinto, the Grand Master of the Knights of Malta and St John.

In Rome he married the beautiful Lorenza Feliciani, who was to share his adventures and aid his charades with her glamour. From there he travelled to Holstein where he met another medical meddler and occultist, the Count St Germain.

In 1776 he arrived in Strasbourg where he started treating the poor for free, while peddling cures to the rich and making it known that he had discovered the Elixir of Youth. To visibly demonstrate the power of this elixir to rejuvenate people he declared that Lorenza was the living proof, since she was over 60 years of age, yet looked 20. She was in fact only 20 years of age. As a result, his reputation then preceded him wherever he went. Next he went to London where he established the cult of Egyptian Freemasonry, calling himself the Grand Cophta. It was a short stay, however, as some of his double-dealing was discovered and he was forced to flee to Paris.

There the Count of Cagliostro's claims became more and more outrageous. He claimed that he was so old that he had met various historical figures like Julius Caesar and Alexander the Great, and that he had been in Rome when it burned during the reign of the emperor Nero. He practiced quack medicine and necromancy, in which he held spectacular séances during which he would claim to communicate with the dead. Not only that, but through his communication with the spirits he claimed to be able to foretell the future. People flocked to him to have their fortunes told.

He also became intimately acquainted with Cardinal de Rohan and was implicated in the Affair of the Diamond Necklace in 1785. This was to be one of the causes of the French Revolution. For his part in it he was thrown into the Bastille for six months before being expelled from France, prior to which he predicted that the Bastille would one day soon be razed to the ground. Amazingly, it was one of his predictions that proved to be true, for it was indeed razed during the Terror in 1789.

At Basel he was visited by Johann Caspar Lavater, whom we shall meet in Chapter 4 Physiognomy. Lavater seemed to be impressed with Cagliostro and did not read anything of his duplicitous character in his face.

In 1789 he travelled again to Rome, duly falling foul of the Inquisition. In 1790 he was tried and found guilty of practising freemasonry and sorcery. He was incarcerated first in San Angelo and then in San Leone in the duchy of Urbino, where he died. The details of his death are not known, but one theory is that he was strangled. Another is that he somehow escaped and retired to die peacefully away from the limelight. The latter is highly improbable, given his lifelong craving for publicity and adulation.

Lorenza entered a nunnery and spent the rest of her life atoning for her adventurous life of deception with Cagliostro.

3

WATER, ELECTRICITY AND FRESH AIR

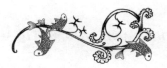

As to diseases, make a habit of two things – to help, or at least, to do no harm.
Air Waters and Places, Hippocrates (460–377 BC)

Cleanliness is next to godliness.

Reverend John Wesley (1703–91)

Hippocrates, the father of medicine, taught that a physician should get to know the air, the wind, the water and the very nature of the soil and the sort of plants that grew in and around the city to which the itinerant physician would go. It was good wholesome advice based on sound reasoning. Essentially it was the bedrock of public health medicine. Yet as we saw in the last chapter there were always medical meddlers prepared to take a thread of truth or good sense and weave from it an entire blanket of falsehood and promises of cures for all ills. In the Victorian Age of Credulity many would seize upon scientific advances and establish a lucrative edifice of medical nonsense.

At the same time, as we shall see, many believed wholeheartedly that they were peddling truth.

AIR AND GASES

The eighteenth century saw the discovery of many gases, which scientists thought were all variants of air. Joseph Priestley had discovered oxygen, although he had mistakenly called it 'dephlogisticated air', since he was a firm believer in the phlogiston theory. This had been the dominant theory of combustion in the early days of chemistry. Adherents to it thought that when something burned or rusted, it released a substance called phlogiston into the air and a physical residue of ash or rust. The French scientist Antoine-Laurent de Lavoisier (1743–94) disproved this and demonstrated clearly that the gas 'oxygen', as he called it, was needed for combustion to take place.

Priestley went on to discover ten more gases, including ammonia, sulphur dioxide and nitrous oxide. Henry Cavendish (1731–1810) discovered hydrogen and others steadily added to the list.

Yet because they were all considered akin to air it was inevitable that someone would try to see whether they could be adapted to the treatment of illness and disease.

DR THOMAS BEDDOES AND PNEUMATIC MEDICINE

Dr Thomas Beddoes (1760–1808) was one such genuine believer. In fact, Dr Thomas Beddoes was a believer in many things in his time and in a way he was a catalyst for some of the spectacular advances that would occur in Victorian science and medicine. His advocacy of what he called 'pneumatic medicine' was not one of them.

This is not to denigrate Thomas Beddoes, for he was a good man, an educated man and a philanthropist. Like many cultured men of his era he studied both medicine and chemistry. He studied medicine in Edinburgh then moved ever southwards, to Bath, then Oxford and London, before settling in Bristol.

Some of his ideas sound decidedly odd. One such was his observation that butchers rarely suffered from consumption. When he asked some of them he received the reply that the inhalation of the odours in the slaughterhouse was health-giving! He pondered on this and concluded that the air from the lungs of beasts may be the key and so he actually introduced windows into his clinics through which cattle could poke their heads and breathe upon the ill. Some patients, however, were not so happy about the smell of dung that they were also forced to endure.

When he settled in Bristol he set up the Pneumatic Institute for Inhalation Gas Therapy in nearby Clifton. He firmly believed that the various gases that chemists were discovering were just variants of air and that each gas had the potential to heal. Carbon dioxide had been used to treat consumption, as the disease tuberculosis was then known. Beddoes planned to extend the range and use hydrogen and others.

One of the first patients that he treated was the young daughter of the inventor James Watt, who did have tuberculosis. Unfortunately, she had probably been too ill already and soon succumbed to her illness. Yet James Watt had faith in Beddoes and designed various pieces of apparatus that could be used to deliver gases to patients.

He decided that the institute needed a chemist to help him and, as it happened, the young man that he appointed was the 20-year-old Humphrey Davy. This was fortuitous for it gave Davy the opportunity to develop his skills as a chemist. Soon Davy was inhaling gases that he produced in the laboratory. One of these was nitrous oxide, which he found was quite intoxicating. Not only that, but on one occasion he was suffering from toothache and he discovered that inhaling the gas actually gave pain relief. Strangely enough, although he was working in a purported medical institute, no one realised the potential that laughing gas would have. It fell to an American dentist to discover this fact forty-odd years later.

Davy soon left for greater things than those that were offered by Thomas Beddoes. He became interested in electricity and electrolysis and moved to the Royal Institution in London. As for Tomas Beddoes, his ideas about pneumatic medicine all came to nothing. His vision of supplying every household with an apparatus that would manufacture all of the needed medicinal gases failed and he died a disillusioned man.

ANAESTHESIA

Surgery in the early Victorian era was just as painful a process as it ever had been. The use of nitrous oxide had been suggested by Humphrey Davy, but he did not have a powerful enough voice and he was not a medical man. It was only really used at social 'revels' by the leisured classes.

In 1824 Dr Henry Hill Hickman (1801–30), a young Shropshire country doctor, had followed Dr Beddoes' ideas of inhaling gases and experimented on animals. He induced the state of what he called 'suspended animation' in these animals by making them inhale carbon dioxide gas. He then operated upon them in a seemingly painless manner. He advocated that it should be tried on humans, but his suggestion evoked ridicule. Indeed, an article in *The Lancet* totally derided his work under the title 'Surgical Humbug'.

Hickman did not leave it there, but took his ideas to France, where he obtained a hearing and actually read a paper to King Charles X. The paper was then forwarded to the Academie Royale de Medicine, but once again nothing came of it.

In fact, carbon dioxide would induce such a state, but it would also induce panic attacks in humans. Worse still, it could be fatal! The idea of using gas, however, albeit in this case the wrong one, did have merit as a means of inducing a sleep-like state.

By 1831 three anaesthetic agents had been discovered. They were chloroform, ether and nitrous oxide. In 1842 in the United States, Dr Crawford W. Long (1815–78) performed three minor operations on humans using ether. Two years later, a dentist, Dr Horace Wells (1815–48), used ether on himself and had one of his own teeth removed.

A friend of his, Dr William T.G. Morton (1819–68), used it to perform surgery in a demonstration to other doctors. It was the beginning of a new era for surgery and the name 'anaesthesia' was devised by Oliver Wendell Holmes.

Back in Britain, James Simpson started to use chloroform, which was less irritant and more pleasing to be given. He advocated giving it to mothers during labour, but met with opposition from the Calvinist Church, who said that it was natural for a woman to endure pain to bring a child into the world. This view was quickly scotched, however, when in 1853 Dr John Snow (1813–58) gave chloroform to Queen Victoria herself when she had her son Leopold. He repeated this in 1857 when she gave birth to her daughter Beatrice.

ELECTRICITY

Electricity was in the air in Victorian times. That is to say that the discoveries about electricity that had been made in the previous century had opened up whole new areas of research. The Italian Luigi Galvani (1737–98), an anatomist and professor of obstetrics at Bologna University, had performed experiments on frogs' legs and discovered that electricity could make them twitch. Then Alessandro Volta (1745–1827), a professor of physics at Pavia University, invented the first battery, the voltaic pile.

It seemed that this was a power that could have immense benefit in medicine – as well as great potential for wealth in the hands of the medical meddlers.

JOHN WESLEY AND ETHEREAL FIRE

The name of John Wesley (1703–91) is forever associated with Methodism, which he founded along with his younger brother Charles Wesley. He was an Anglican minister but found himself banned from many pulpits because his religious views were considered radical. He therefore travelled extensively, both in England and America, preaching in open areas to the poor whom he often found to be excluded from churches. In America he railed against the practice of slavery.

Not only did he believe that he was called to help people with their spiritual needs, he also wrote about medicine and how people could use self-help techniques when they were ill. His book *Primitive Physick* was published in 1747 and was widely sold and used.

John Wesley and his ethereal fire or electrotherapy machine.

In that same year he saw for the first time an exhibition of galvanism, or the use of electric batteries called Leyden jars to create shocks. Wesley was quick to grasp the opportunities that this amazing power, which he called 'ethereal fire', could hold. He became a devotee of electrotherapy and began using it to treat the poor on his travels and in a special free dispensary that he established. In 1759 he wrote *The Desideratum, or Electricity made plain and useful.*

Wesley subscribed to the theory that ethereal fire, as they knew electricity, caused capillaries to dilate and that it released all manner of blockages that were causing disease.

Soon ethereal fire was being used to give shocks to people to cure them of arthritis and rheumatism, epilepsy, blindness, paralysis, back pain, sciatica and that cursed affliction of the spirits, melancholia. So successful were his treatments that other dispensaries were established and Wesley's reputation as a healer soared.

Although one would have to say that this was medical meddling on a grand scale, for he had no medical qualifications or credentials whatsoever, many of the conditions that he treated may have been amenable to electrical shocks. Certainly his use of it in melancholia may have been one of the only effective treatments at that time.

VICTORIAN ELECTROTHERAPY

The Victorians were ingenious at constructing machines and gadgets. There was something awe-inspiring about medical machines with wires, rotating parts and cylinders and flasks that sparked and produced shocks. Doctors all over the country invested in electrotherapy machines to treat everything from headaches to piles. Indeed, a common treatment for piles was called 'anal faradism', which involved the insertion of a rod into the rectum followed by an electrical discharge to singe the piles. It must have been excruciating.

All manner of belts, straps, rings and supports, which could be 'charged', were devised. They all had a dramatic effect, since they would produce a sensation that people could feel, and since they felt it so strongly it would be likely to produce a strong placebo effect. This is not to say, however, that any beneficial effect would be purely placebic, since we know today that various types of electrical stimulation can be helpful in the management of pain. Transcutaneous Electrical Nerve Stimulation, or TNS, is such a method commonly used today.

Of less certain effect, however, would be the 'Galvanic Spectacles', which were invented and patented by Judah Moses of Hartford, United States, in 1868. A British patent for a similar invention was granted to John Leighton in 1888. These consisted of a spectacles frame with a zinc plate and a chrome plate which settled over the bridge of the nose, with leads that attached to a small galvanic battery. A discharge of electricity was thought to stimulate the optic nerve, which they proposed would improve the eyesight. Some users of the galvanic spectacles even suggested that it would clear sinusitis and cure the common cold.

Lots of other devices were manufactured and used by doctors, medical meddlers on the make and members of the public, who bought them to treat their families. Since they seemed to be scientific, they were thought to be effective and a sign that one was keeping up to date with the great discoveries of Victorian science.

In Paris in 1853 Dr Guillaume Duchenne published an account of his success with electricity in various conditions. His work *A Treatise on Localised Electrization and its Application to Pathology and Therapeutics* was to prove influential in medical circles.

Doctors working in the medical asylums of the day had virtually no effective treatments. Patients were physically restrained and there was no drug that could help psychotic states or the harrowing condition of melancholia. Electrotherapy seemed to offer some help, even if no one knew how it worked. There were three types of electricity that they could use: galvanism, which produced a direct current; faradism, or an induced current; and static electricity given directly or charged in a Leyden jar. However, despite initial promise and continued use during the Victorian era the results were quite disappointing and eventually it fell into disuse. It was not reintroduced until 1938 when Cerletti and Bini introduced a very specific therapeutic use of electricity in the technique of Electro-Convulsive Therapy, or ECT, in which electricity was applied to one or both hemispheres of the brain in order to induce a convulsion.

Dr Golding Bird, a physician at Guy's Hospital in London, was concerned about the proliferation of electrical gadgets and their unsystematic use, especially by unqualified people whom he considered to be quacks. While he thought that electrotherapy had a place, he thought that it should only be used on neurological conditions. One can see his logic, since he perceived neurological conditions to be the result of damaged nerves, which were unable to conduct electrical activity properly. Electrotherapy could 'flush' them out, so to speak.

Other doctors were not as rigid and thought that electrotherapy had a legitimate place in the treatment of rheumatic and arthritic conditions. Indeed, it was in this area that its use would thrive all through the Victorian era and well into the twentieth century. Even today, in the twenty-first century, it has a place in many painful conditions, when used under the guidance of appropriately trained practitioners.

WATER

The use of baths and various types of water treatments had been used for many hundreds of years. Bronze Age metal tubing has been found at St Moritz in Switzerland, the site of natural hot springs. The Minoans built great palaces complete with rudimentary plumbed baths at Knossos in Crete as long ago as the second millennium BC. Similarly, in the Indus valley pre-Aryans built highly civilised cities at Harappa and Mohendjo-daro, using a grid system containing piped water, sewage conduits, a network of wells and both public and private baths.

The ancient Greeks embraced bathing as both a pleasurable and a healthy activity. Greek physicians extolled the virtues of different types of bath and advised upon the use of oils in the water and for anointing before one dried off. In the first century AD a Greek physician, Aesclepiades of Bithynia, attained great fame in Rome where he founded the Methodical School of Medicine. He advocated using contraries (medicines which were contrary to the symptoms of illness), as well as generous diets, strenuous exercise and bathing. It is likely that it was he who was responsible for introducing the Roman ideal of frequent baths, and indirectly responsible for the enthusiasm with which the Romans built baths near medicinal springs and wells.

As the Roman Empire spread across Europe, spas were established at Aix-le-Bains and Vicy in France (respectively called by them Aquae Gratianae and Aqua Calidae), and at Wiesbaden and Baden Baden in Germany (respectively Aquae Mattiacae and Aurelia Aquensis), then at Bath in England (Aquae Sulis).

The Romans developed the building of baths into a fine art, thanks to their skill at engineering and their use of the hypocaust system of underground heating. A typical Roman bath house would have several rooms, through which the bather went in turn. The first room was the *frigidarium*, which was the unheated cold room in which they changed. There the bather cooled down and perhaps even took a cold bath or shower. After that he went into the *tepidarium*, the warm room which was the first of the rooms to receive some heat from the hypocaust. Here the bather had oils rubbed into the skin to start the process of opening the pores. After the acclimatisation had begun, he moved through to the *caldarium*, the hot room where the air was really hot and humid by virtue of a steam tank attached to the hypocaust. Indeed, so hot was this room that the floor could be too hot for the bare feet and one was obliged to wear thick wooden sandals.

In the *caldarium* the bather could wash his face at the central cold water *labrum*, a basin atop a pedestal, then lounge and chat on one of the benches and couches, while the perspiration and skin residues would be scraped from him with a smooth comb called a *strigil*. That done, he could move to the hottest room, the *laconicum*, before returning to the *frigidarium* for a further cold water plunge and a dry off.

Healing wells were used by people all over Europe from prehistoric times. The Celts and other peoples considered them to be sacred places and often erected shrines by them. When Christianity spread across the continent these healing wells were blessed and became incorporated into the Church as holy wells.

In the sixteenth and seventeenth centuries many of these holy wells became very important as various doctors began to extol the virtues of taking the waters. Among these was Dr William Turner, who in 1562 published *A booke of the nature and properties of the bathes of England ... and other countries*. Before long the era of the spa towns had begun (all named after Spa in Belgium, the original centre). At these centres people would come to drink the waters and bathe.

HYDROPATHY COMES INTO ITS OWN

In the early nineteenth century Vincent Priessnitz (1799–1851) formalised the various treatments that had been used into a system of medicine that he called 'hydropathy', from *hydro* meaning 'water' and *pathos* meaning 'suffering'; implying that water could be used to relieve illness.

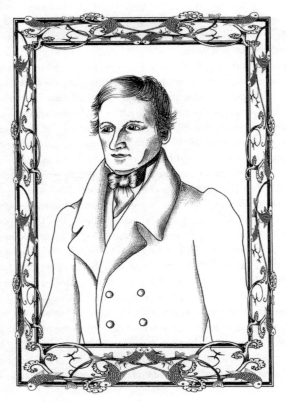

Vincent Priessnitz.

Priessnitz was born into a peasant farming family in Silesia, which was later to become Jesenic in Czechoslovakia. Apparently he was a keen observer of all wildlife as a boy and had noticed how injured or unwell animals or birds would stop eating and take themselves off to water where they would drink and bathe. From this he reasoned that water was in some way healing. Then, as a young man, he injured his leg and was disappointed when it failed to respond to medical treatment. He accordingly devised a means of treating it himself using water in various ways. From this personal success he began treating other people and soon established his system of using cold water upon the patient in the form of baths, sprays, showers, cold wraps, sponges and rubs. It became known as the 'cold water cure', since no other medicines or drugs were given and nothing was added to the water. He did, however, also advocate abstemiousness, wholesome diet and exercise, all of which would certainly have helped.

His reputation spread like wildfire and patients flocked from all over Europe to see him. In the year 1839 alone, it is recorded that among his clientele he saw twenty-two princes and princesses, one duke, one duchess, 149 counts and countesses, eighty-eight barons and baronesses ... and many, many more of lesser rank!

Doctors also went to learn his methods and carried the practice of hydropathy across the world. Two English physicians, Dr James Wilson (1807–67) and Dr James Manby Gully (1808–83), established a hydropathic centre in Malvern, England in 1842. Others followed suit and in the following decades a succession of hydropathic hospitals and hotels were established throughout the British Isles.

The Malvern Water Cure Centre extended Priessnitz's ideas beyond that of just using various applications of cold water. They used homoeopathy and advised upon taking the Malvern spring water medicinally. The establishment soon became famous and the two doctors became nationally celebrated figures. Accordingly, the great and famous beat a path to their centre for treatment. Among those who apparently attended were Charles Darwin, Charles Dickens, Florence Nightingale, Lord Tennyson and Thomas Carlyle. How successful their respective treatments were is not clear, although Darwin wrote that he was sceptical to say the least.

In January 1867 Dr Wilson felt unwell, which he attributed to overwork, and went for a rest to Ben Rhydding in Yorkshire, another health centre renowned for its waters. There he ordered a tepid bath to be drawn for him, but tragically he was found dead some time later half-dressed in a chair beside the bath which had turned cold.

Dr Gully continued in his successful practice in Malvern. Sadly, towards the end of his life he was involved in a scandal that would blight his reputation ever after. He retired from his practice and left Malvern in 1873. He met a young woman called Florence Ricardo, whom he began an affair with. They travelled to Kissingen in Germany and Florence became pregnant. Dr Gully apparently performed an abortion after which they parted. Soon after this Florence met and married Charles Bravo, whom she married in 1875. This incensed Dr Gully when he received a letter from a friend informing him of the marriage.

A few months afterwards Charles Bravo died from poisoning. An inquest was held at which Dr Gully was called to testify. Both he and Florence had been suspected of the poisoning, although nothing came of the case. The medical societies to which he belonged felt that the association with the case brought the profession into disrepute and his name was removed from their membership. He died in 1883.

HOMOEOPATHY

In the eighteenth century Dr Samuel Hahnemann (1755–1843) developed the system of medicine known as homoeopathy, based upon the principle of using 'like to cure like'. In other words he used diluted and potentised remedies made from substances that produced similar symptoms to the condition the patient was suffering from. Thus a remedy made from onions, which cause streaming eyes and nose, could be given to treat a cold with such symptoms, or a remedy from nettles to treat someone with a nettle rash.

Hahnemann had formulated his ideas in a book called *Organon of Rational Healing* in 1810. It subsequently went through six editions, it being generally known as the *Organon*.

Homoeopathy was controversial in Hahnemann's own day and it has never been free of its sceptics. Nevertheless, it spread across the world and was immensely popular in the Victorian era, as indeed it still is in the twenty-first century. Many of the doctors who were involved in hydropathic practice were also homoeopathic physicians. Indeed, the two approaches had a similar philosophy.

NATURE

The philosophical link between hydropathy and homoeopathy was their non-drug approach. This was further developed in the mid-nineteenth century with the rise of the nature cure.

The nature cure movement developed the idea that illness was the result of an accumulation of toxins within the body. The aim of medicine, according to some doctors, was to encourage the body to discharge or expel these toxins, which would permit the body to rebalance itself. In other words, nature knows best and the physician should merely try to assist nature to achieve the cure.

Priessnitz had been extremely influential with his hydropathic approach. At about the same time an Austrian practitioner, Johannes Schroth (1798–1856), set up a clinic which also advised the water cure and a dry food diet.

Pastor Sebastian Kneipp (1827–97), a Bavarian priest and a pupil of Priessnitz, advocated hot and cold water cures, claiming that he had cured his own tuberculosis by bathing in the River Danube. He also advocated the use of various herbs and oft repeated this aphorism: 'Many people died while the herbs that could have saved them grow on their graves.'

In the United States a number of conventionally trained doctors like Dr John Harvey Kellog and Dr Henry Lindlahr took up the methods and formulated them into a system called 'naturopathy', which drew on hydropathy, homeopathy, herbalism and nutrition.

In Britain Dr Henry Allinson (1858–1918) advocated exercise, not smoking, and taking a diet of wholesome food, especially with wholegrain bread. His opposition to the use of strong drugs and to vaccination, however, were to result in him getting in trouble with the General Medical Council, which struck him off the register. Despite this he continued his advocacy of a natural lifestyle and the consumption of wholegrain bread, such as could be made from the flour that his own mill produced. His name lives on today associated with the family flour business.

The nature cure attracted its critics, who lampooned the excessive use of enemas and such activities as running around without shoes in order to soak up the natural dew from the morning grass.

TEMPERANCE

Running in tandem with the nature cure, indeed, often seen as part of it, was the temperance movement.

William Hogarth splendidly depicts the drunkenness of the eighteenth century in his famous etchings of Gin Lane and Beer Alley. The thing was that water had never been seen to be particularly safe and so much of the population was addicted to wine, spirits, beer or porter.

In 1854 Dr John Snow, the physician who had administered chloroform to Queen Victoria, proved that cholera was a water-borne disease when he traced an outbreak in London back to the use of a communal well in Broad Street, Soho. Snow removed the handle of the well and the number of cases rapidly fell. The well had been receiving infected leakage from a sewer.

Social reformers had seen drinking alcohol as a huge problem that kept people in poverty, drove crime and caused death through accidents and drink-related disease. In 1830 the first temperance society was formed in England in the city of Bradford. Linked with religion, workers strove to get drinkers to abstain and 'take the pledge'.

To go 'teetotal' is a phrase that drifted into common parlance. Rather than having anything to do with tea, however, as many people imagine it, the word was inadvertently coined by a reformed drinker by the name of Dick Turner in Preston in 1833. He declared in a speech delivered in a rich Yorkshire accent that: 'I'll have nowt to do with this moderation; I'll be reet down and out tee-tee-total for ever!'

Although some doctors did follow the temperance movement they were not in the majority. The reason was that so many medicines were prepared with some alcoholic content, or indeed using alcohol as an integral part of the prescription. That is not surprising considering that many of the medicines were probably quite ineffective. The main effect could have been the numbing action of the alcohol, the suppression of inhibitions and the lightening of the mood that a little alcohol seems to produce.

THE MEDICAL ACT OF 1858

As will have been evident in the sojourn through medical history and medical meddling thus far, anyone could practice medicine with or without a degree or qualification. In 1858 parliament passed the Medical Act in order to regulate the practice of medicine and surgery in the British Isles. It created a register of qualified practitioners and a body that would regulate those practitioners. This was the General Medical Council, which is still operational today.

Most of the 1858 act has been repealed and replaced by the Medical Act of 1983, but even this is under review. From 2011 all doctors practicing in the UK were issued with a licence to practice medicine. From 2012 a process of revalidation will take place, in which the license to practice will have to be reapplied for every five years.

None of these acts, however, have ever stopped the medical meddlers.

4

PHYSIOGNOMY

I maintain what is manifest to every eye, however inexperienced, that there is beauty, or deformity, in the features of the face.

Essays on Physiognomy, 1775–78
Johann Caspar Lavater

The Victorians were quite obsessed with character and with methods of assessing it. It was very much tied in with concepts of health and medicine for there was still a widely held belief that the temperament one was born with could predispose one to various types of illness.

In the Victorian era physiognomy, or the study of character through analysis of facial features, was enthusiastically practiced by professionals and amateurs alike. People assessed the worth of others by the shape of their faces, the prominence or otherwise of ears, nose and chin, the slant of eyebrows, the twist of the mouth or the readiness with which the face took up a particular expression. Marriages, business alliances and the hiring and firing of workers could be based upon the study of a face. How scientific can such a study be? It is perhaps germane to consider a little anecdote concerning one of the most famous scientists of all time, the man whose life's work would involve a study of nature in general and of his fellow man in particular.

NATURALIST WANTED!

In 1830 Robert Fitzroy (1805–65) was given the position of captain of HMS *Beagle* after his predecessor, Captain Pringle-Stocks, had shot himself following a bout of melancholia occasioned by loneliness.

At his own expense Fitzroy determined to take the ship on an expedition to Tierra del Fuego because he intended to take three young Indians home. He had previously brought a party of four Fuegan natives back to England with the intention of educating them so that they could return and spread the knowledge that they had been given. Sadly, one of the four had died of smallpox, so his voyage may have been prompted by some degree of guilt.

Since HMS *Beagle* was a hydrographic survey vessel, Fitzroy advertised for a naturalist to accompany him. One of the applicants was a young 22-year-old divinity graduate from Cambridge by the name of Charles Darwin. Fitzroy happened to be an enthusiastic student of physiognomy and although he liked Darwin well enough he considered that his nose was too short. This led him to believe that he would not be robust enough to endure the long sea voyage that he estimated would almost take five years. He therefore appointed another applicant.

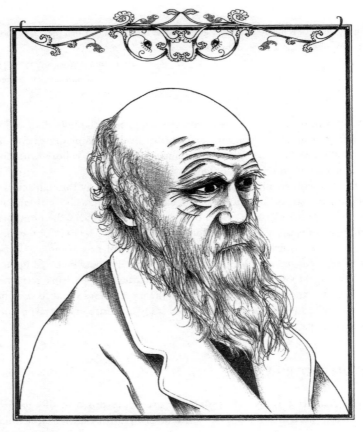

Charles Darwin.

One wonders if things may have been different had the first-choice candidate not turned down the position. The voyage of the *Beagle* was very important in shaping the young naturalist's ideas. Perhaps Darwin would not have developed his theory of evolution, arguably the greatest scientific discovery in the history of mankind, had he not visited the Galapagos Islands with Fitzroy and seen the flora and fauna that had evolved in that idyllic part of the world which was so devoid of natural predators. As it was, Darwin went on to write *On the Origin of Species*, one of the great books of the world that was to have such a profound effect upon science and the way that we view the planet and our place in it.

Indeed, it may have been touch and go and it could be said that evolution only had it by a short nose.

PHYSIOGNOMY

The study of the face as a means of working out character and temperament had been practiced as long ago as ancient Greece. Hippocrates (460–377 BC), the father of medicine, referred to facial features and coined the term 'physiognomia' – from *physis*, meaning 'nature', and *gnomon*, meaning 'judgement' or 'interpretation' – in his book on *Epidemics*. He had observed that various features occur in people when they have an illness. In fact, the *Hippocratic facies* is a description of the face that occurs in many debilitating diseases, whereby eyes get sunken, the cheeks become concave, the lips relax and the complexion goes leaden. It is still found in any modern textbook of medicine.

Aristotle (384–322 BC) wrote a treatise on it entitled *Physiognomics*, in which he discussed the face and expressions as they relate to the way in which people thought and behaved. In the middle ages it was called 'visnomy' and was considered a suitable study for people of learning and refinement.

In the early seventeenth century Dr Robert Fludd (1574–1637), a physician, astrologer, mathematician, philosopher and occultist, had postulated that there was a link between the universe, the macrocosm and man, the microcosm. He was a man of great intelligence and ingenuity who postulated that it was possible to build various types of perpetual motion machine. Indeed, in his musings about the human body he suspected that the blood actually circulated around the body, rather like a perpetual motion machine, its only limit being death.

In Fludd's time medicine was still heavily influenced by astrology, the Doctrine of Humors and all manner of archaic and arcane knowledge. Chiromancy, the art of reading character and fortunes from the hand, was widely practiced. One can understand this since the way that an individual uses their hands is unique to them as individuals. It would seem quite logical to postulate that the development of the hand would reflect one's character. Indeed, in the *Art of Chiromancy*, published in 1545, there are very clear instructions for interpreting the various lines on the hand, relating them to the different planets, and relating them to character and future tendencies.

Robert Fludd attempted to do the same with the face and the head. He stated that the face is divided into three 'worlds'. The forehead was related to the divine world; the areas around the nose and eyes represented the physical world; and the mouth and chin linked with the material world. The front of the head related to the thinking part of man and the back of the head was where memories were stored.

Exactly how he came to deduce these various connections is not clear, yet in an age when superstition and a belief in the occult were rampant, it was a clear attempt to lift medicine into the scientific realm and provide a model of the mind.

Sir Thomas Browne (1605–82) was a physician and antiquary who had studied medicine in France, Italy and Holland. He gained a medical degree from the University of Leyden in 1633 and from Oxford in 1637. He then began practising in Norwich and soon built up a successful practice, which allowed him to maintain contact with his fellow antiquaries and scientists of the day, even throughout the tumultuous period of the English Civil War.

He was a prolific author and a student of nature. In 1643 his famous work *Religio Medici* was published. This book (*The Religion of a Doctor*) had in fact been written for his own amusement, but somehow a copy was published in Latin in 1642, containing some segments that had not been written by Browne. He felt compelled to publish the authorised version. The text is essentially about faith, but it covers a whole range of subjects including alchemy, philosophy, astrology and physiognomy. It became a huge bestseller across the whole of Europe. In 1671 he was knighted by King Charles II when he visited Norwich.

Browne believed that physiognomy was a powerful tool that permitted one to read one's fellow men:

> … there is surely a Physiognomy, which those experienced and Master Mendicants observe, whereby they instantly discover a merciful aspect, and will single out a face wherein they spy the signatures and marks of Mercy. For there are mystically in our faces certain Characters which carry in them the motto of our Souls, wherein he that cannot read A. B. C. may read our natures.

Not only that, he wrote that physiognomy could be extended to the whole of nature:

> I hold moreover that there is a Phytognomy, or Physiognomy, not only of Men, but of Plants and Vegetables; and in every one of them some outward figures which hang as signs or bushes of their inward forms. The Finger of God hath left an Inscription upon all His works, not graphical or composed of Letters, but of their several forms, constitutions, parts, and operations, which, aptly joyned together, do make one word that doth express their natures.

JOHANN CASPAR LAVATER

Sir Thomas Browne's *Religio Medici* had a profound influence on the Swiss poet, orator, essayist and Pastor Johann Caspar Lavater (1741–1801), who was to become the main advocate of physiognomy.

Lavater professed to be able to 'read the mind's construction in the face'. Essentially, he taught that the overall shape of the face related to the temperament of the individual and that the individual features revealed the character.

The head to the eyebrows revealed the intellectual ability of the person. The nose and cheeks showed their moral tendencies. The mouth and chin would show the animal characteristics and instincts. Everything would then be amalgamated in the study of the eyes.

In his book *Essays on Physiognomy*, which he wrote between 1789 and 1793, he included over 400 plates showing different features and expressions, and outlined the methods to be followed for making an analysis. He illustrated his essays with depictions of famous figures from history, and of prominent people of his time. Philosophers from Aristotle to Zeno, the crowned heads of Europe from Charles I of England to Louis XIV of France, the emperors of Rome, the writers of the world and the priests, sages and saints of Christendom, all had their faces analysed and their expressions scrutinised.

Some of Lavater's facial types.

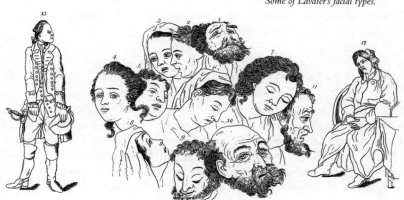

Wit (intelligence) and imagination were two of the key attributes needed by a good physiognomist in his view:

> Imagination is necessary to impress the traits with exactness, so that they may be renewed at leisure; and to range the pictures in the mind as perfectly as if they still were visible, and with all possible order.

By this he meant that one had to use the imagination to see the face and to imagine it falling into different expressions. Many an analysis would be done from a picture or a painting, since this was before the days of photography:

> Wit is indispensable to the physiognomist, that he may easily perceive the resemblances that exist between objects. Thus, for example, he sees a head or forehead possessed of certain characteristic marks. These marks present themselves to his imagination, and wit discovers to what they are similar.

He also taught that a physiognomist must be an artist, able to render the form of the face on paper. He must be knowledgeable about anatomy, physiology and about nature. He very much saw it as being a higher calling, a means of understanding the person's nature, their character and their mind.

He also gave 100 rules that would become promulgated as absolute indicators of character and temperament. It was one such rule that may almost have prevented Charles Darwin from sailing on the *Beagle*:

Rule XLIV

Nose

> A hundred flat snub-noses may be met with in men of great prudence, discretion, and abilities of various kinds. But when the nose is very small, and has an unappropriate upper lip; or when it exceeds a certain degree of flatness, no other feature or lineament of the countenance can rectify it.

MOUNTEBANK PHYSIOGNOMISTS

One can see how such character reading could potentially have dire consequences for those people whose faces literally did not fit. There was also huge potential for charlatanry. Indeed, many mountebanks incorporated physiognomy, which sounded wonderfully scientific, into their repertoire of skills. At fairs, markets and all manner of gatherings itinerant face-readers would give the people what the people wanted – a good character reading with the promise of good fortune. All that it required was the handing over of silver, as one would to any authentic looking fortune-teller, and have one's face read.

The Vagrancy Act of 1744,[2] however, made this a dangerous thing to profess skill at. The penalty was a whipping or six months in jail.

---

2. The Act 17 George II. C. 5 This was the Vagrancy Act. The method of recording acts at that time related to the year of the monarch's reign, hence the seventeenth year of King George II's reign.

VICTORIAN PHYSIOGNOMY

Lavater's ideas about physiognomy were not just taken up by rogues and charlatans, but were taken seriously by the medical profession during the Victorian age. It was a highly plausible theory and it smacked of having a basic scientific truth.

Mental illness was poorly understood and there was no proper theory of psychology or model of the workings of the mind that could be used in order to make a firm diagnosis of any mental condition. Basically, there was sanity and insanity. To be diagnosed as insane meant that one could be incarcerated in one of the lunatic asylums, in some instances a far worse fate than being sent to prison.

In the last of his series of eight lithographs that made up *The Rake's Progress*, William Hogarth gives us an insight into an eighteenth-century asylum at Bedlam. Inmates were kept in chains and people paid to go and see the patients, as one would pay to visit a fair or see a play being performed. Although he painted this in 1735, the treatment of people in asylums did not improve until the very end of the century. Then Dr Philippe Pinel, the superintendent at the Bicetre Asylum in Paris, had the chains struck off his patients and a more humane approach was adopted. It took time for this to happen in Britain and Robin Gardiner Hill, the superintendent of the Lincoln Mental Asylum, is credited as the first person in England to abolish restraints.

In 1840 Sir Alexander Morison (1799–1866), the physician to the Bethlehem Hospital, published *The Physiognomy of Mental Diseases*. This was a series of portraits of 'lunatics'. It was the direct application of Lavater's work to medicine. It was a highly influential piece of work which was rapidly adopted as a means by which doctors could base their diagnoses.

In 1852 Hugh Welch Diamond (1809–66), the resident superintendent of the female department of the Surrey County Lunatic Asylum, assembled a series of photographic portraits of patients to illustrate the various types of insanity. He then presented a paper to the Royal Society in 1852, setting out three functions of the new science of photography in the treatment of the mentally ill. These were:

> To record the appearance and expressions of patients with different mental conditions, based upon the principles of physiognomy.
>
> To use photographs as a means of identification for readmission and treatment.
>
> To enable comparison images to be made showing progress with treatment.

Diamond became known as the father of psychiatric photography.

THE LUNATIC PANIC

There was always a great fear of mental illness in the Victorian age. A fear of becoming insane and a fear of those who were mentally ill. As mentioned earlier, the penalty of being diagnosed insane was to be incarcerated in the asylum. This fear reached a peak in the years 1858–59, and it centred on Dr John Conolly, a noted psychiatrist and professor of medicine at University College, London.

Conolly had a brilliant and successful career, having adopted a non-restraint policy while he was the superintendent at Hanwell Asylum. In 1858 he wrote a series of essays on *The Physiognomy of Insanity*, drawing on the photographs of Hugh Welch Diamond and others to illustrate his theories.

His reputation nosedived in 1858, however, following his commitment of the novelist Rosina Bulwer Lytton (1802–82). She was a famous novelist in her own right and renowned as the Irish beauty who had married Edward Bulwer Lytton, later Lord Lytton, himself a famed novelist and politician. Their marriage had not been a happy one and they were legally separated in 1836. She despised his political aspirations and when he stood as a parliamentary candidate for Hertfordshire in 1858 she heckled him. This resulted in her being restrained and quickly declared insane. Dr John Conolly certified her at the request of her husband, possibly for a large fee, and she was admitted to Wyke House, a private asylum.

There was a public outcry and the case featured prominently in the press. As a result, she was released from the asylum after a few weeks, having been declared cured by Dr Conolly. Other cases were cited and it was alleged that he had wrongfully committed several other people. Indeed, it set off the Lunatic Panic of 1858–59 in which people developed a great fear of the ease with which doctors could apparently remove people from society and deprive them of their rights and their freedom.

Indeed, the whole episode and the problem of the commitment of people to asylums on very flimsy grounds, like physiognomy, became the subject of the 1863 novel *Hard Cash* by Charles Reade, serialised in Charles Dickens's *All the Year Round Magazine*. In it the protagonist is cheated out of his inheritance by his father and committed to an asylum on payment of a fee by his father. The doctor is a thinly disguised version of Dr Conolly.

CHARLES DARWIN'S WORK

The great naturalist Charles Darwin was no lover of physiognomy, although he did work on expressions himself. Indeed, his 1872 book *Expression of the Emotions in Man and Animals* laid the foundations for 'ethology', the study of behaviour and body language.

He concluded that there are six basic facial expressions common to all humans regardless of their race or place of origin. They are essentially inherited.
They are the emotions of happiness, sadness, fear, surprise, anger and disgust.

THE PICTURE OF DORIAN GRAY

Oscar Wilde (1854–1900), one of the world's greatest writers, was intrigued by cheiromancy (palmistry) and physiognomy, among other abstruse subjects, which he incorporated into his short stories and plays. His novel *The Picture of Dorian Gray*, first serialised in *Lippincott's Magazine* in 1890, is very much based around the ideas of physiognomy, and the way that moral degradation will reflect in the face of the portrait of Dorian Gray. It is probably one of the most accomplished novels of the Victorian age.

Ironically, the decay of the portrait mirrored the decline of physiognomy as the Victorian age came to an end.

5

PHRENOLOGY

I declare that the phrenological system of mental philosophy is as much better than
all other systems as the electric light is better than the tallow dip.

William E. Gladstone (1809–98)

Not to know yourself phrenologically is sure to keep you standing on the Bridge of
Sighs all your life.

Andrew Carnegie (1835–1919)

Related to physiognomy was the study and practice of phrenology. Essentially
it was a system devised by Dr Franz Joseph Gall at the end of the eighteenth
century, which proposed that the shape of the skull mirrored the convolutions of
the brain. The term was derived from the Greek *phren*, meaning 'mind', and *logos*,
meaning 'study of' or 'knowledge'.

From extensive anatomical studies and empirical observation Gall had
concluded that the brain was made up of individual organs or faculties, each
of which represented the various temperaments, emotions, mental abilities and
controlling functions of the body. By assessing the shape of the skull, the size of
its prominences, its lumps and bumps, he came to believe that it was possible to
predict an individual's strengths and weaknesses, their potentials and their failings.

In the Victorian era professional phrenologists set up in consulting rooms like
any medical specialist or general practitioner and made good livings. People
flocked to them to have their heads read, to see what they should be doing with
their lives, and to gain answers in matters of love, business and life in general.
Children were taken to see what path of life they should be groomed for.

It seemed a highly plausible discipline, perfect for the Victorian Age of Credulity.

DR FRANZ JOSEPH GALL (1758–1828)

The majority of the extensive Victorian literature on phrenology talks about its 'discovery' as if it was an absolute truth that had been waiting for mankind to uncover. That in itself is quite fascinating, since it illustrates the absolute conviction of practitioners that it was a science every bit as valid as physics, chemistry or botany.

The discoverer and founder was Franz Joseph Gall, who was born on 9 March 1788 at Tiefenbrunn, a village in the Grand Duchy of Baden in Germany. His father was a merchant and mayor. He was an academically able student, and after a disagreement with his parents about a choice of career (they wanted him to become a priest) he went to Vienna and qualified as a doctor. There he developed a reputation as a physician of promise and was offered the post of Medical Counsellor of State to Emperor Francis I. Surprisingly, he very courteously declined, because he felt that it could interfere with his research.

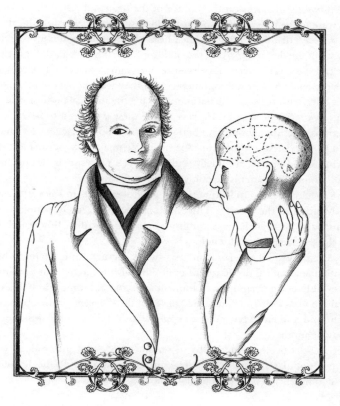

Dr Franz Joseph Gall.

Gall actually had the germ of an idea about the brain and the shape of people's heads when he was a youth, even before he became a medical student. He had noticed that some of his fellow students who had an aptitude for communicating all had rather prominent eyes. He also noticed that others who did not seem as intelligent as himself but who had better memories all seemed to have a wider space between their eyes. Others with a gift for music or art had prominent areas on their heads. All of this, he conjectured, could be due to extra brain development in the areas corresponding to these outward appearances.

He developed these early ideas when he took over the post of physician to a mental asylum in Vienna. There he had ample opportunity to study the heads of the patients. In addition, whenever he heard of anyone having a marked skill or talent he requested permission to examine their head and in many instances also managed to take casts of them. Gradually, he formed his theory that the brain was not just one organ, but an assemblage of a large number of smaller organs, each of which controlled an area of thought or a quality of the person, and which thereby gave the individual their temperament, character and governed their abilities. He outlined twenty-six areas on the surface of the head and called them 'faculties'. These were to form the first of the many phrenological maps of the head.

He believed that by reading people's heads, by examining the prominences or otherwise of the different parts of the skull, he could discover all about the person. In short, it was a very mechanistic science of the mind that fitted extremely well with the sciences of anatomy and medicine as they were known at the time.

After thirty years of study he began informing the medical profession about his findings in a series of lectures. However, since these were seen to be antagonistic to religious teachings about man being made in God's image, his lectures were banned in Austria. Accordingly, in 1802 he left Vienna and went on a lecture tour in Germany and France, eventually settling in Paris where he built up a lucrative practice. Among his patients he numbered ten ambassadors.

In 1819 he was asked to lecture to the medical students in Paris at the request of the Minister of the Interior. These lectures were extremely popular, since he demonstrated his theories by exhibiting brains and skulls. How could anyone doubt the science behind phrenology?

In 1823 he visited England on a six-week lecture tour, during which he performed anatomical dissection of brains. He also brought with him over 300 skulls of different descriptions: of humans and animals, some admirable casts of the brain in wax, over 100 illuminated plates of the different configurations of the cranium, and numerous portraits of people who had distinguished themselves in one way or another.

This was a travelling medical and science show, and phrenology became extremely popular among the medical profession and the public. It seemed to promise so much and it seemed totally plausible.

DR JOHAN GASPAR SPURZHEIM (1776–1832)

A student of Dr Gall's in Vienna, Dr Johan Spurzheim was largely responsible for helping to spread the word about phrenology. An able anatomist, he worked with Gall for many years and dissected brains during lectures while Gall expounded on the findings of the dissections.

In 1814 he settled in England, established a practice and travelled the length and breadth of the land lecturing to doctors and interested lay people. In 1817 he became a licentiate of the Royal College of Physicians. By all accounts he was a cultured, dignified man whose personality attracted many people to phrenology, even those who had at first been steadfast critics.

In 1832 he left for the USA where he gave lectures at Harvard University and Boston. Sadly, he contracted a respiratory illness soon after and died. Yet others had heard his lectures and took up the baton.

THE COMBE BROTHERS

George Combe (1788–1858) was born in Edinburgh and built something of a reputation as a lawyer and philosopher. He attended a lecture by Dr Spurzheim, as a sceptic, but was persuaded by the dissections that he witnessed and the explanations that Spurzheim gave. He thereafter threw himself into the study of the subject and was the first major British phrenologist. In 1820 he founded the Edinburgh Phrenological Society, which would have great influence for the rest of the century. He was a prolific writer and his monographs and papers did much to persuade others to join the phrenological movement.

In 1850 he was invited to Buckingham Palace where he explained the principles of phrenology to Queen Victoria, demonstrating on the heads of the royal children.

Working alongside George was his younger brother, Dr Andrew Combe (1797–1847), an able physician. Indeed, as physician-extraordinary in Scotland to Queen Victoria and consulting physician to the King and Queen of Belgium, his eminence in medicine gave phrenology a sort of legitimacy. He edited *The Edinburgh Phrenological Journal* for over twenty years and defended phrenology before the Royal Medical Society of Edinburgh in 1823.

THE FOWLER BROTHERS

The story of phrenology in the second half of the Victorian era is largely to do with another set of brothers, the remarkable Fowler brothers, originally of New York.

Oscar Squire Fowler (1809–87) studied at Amherst College and was stimulated to study phrenology. He read all of the works of Spurzheim and Combe and adopted it with the zeal of a missionary. He quickly decided that it held truth about the nature of man and that needed to be disseminated. He was joined in this venture by his brother Lorenzo Niles Fowler (1811–96). By 1840 they were reading heads in New York and established a large clientele.

In 1844 they were joined by Samuel R. Wells (1820–75) and set up a publishing house to produce a string of pamphlets, journals and books on phrenology.

Oscar Fowler wrote extensively about phrenology, but also advocated temperance, good nutrition and self-help. He was influential in architectural design and proposed that octagonal style houses instead of rectangular or square ones were better for people to live in. In 1848 he wrote *The Octagon House: A Home For All, or A New, Cheap, Convenient, and Superior Mode of Building*. For a while in the 1850s lots of these were built and the term 'octagon house' refers to the style of building that he proposed. So successful was he in his career and his writing that the town of Fowler in Colorado was named after him.

In 1860 Lorenzo Fowler and Samuel Wells moved to England and began a phrenological practice, gave lectures and set up another publishing company. Lorenzo began producing phrenological busts and soon they were well-nigh ubiquitous throughout the land. Doctors and professional phrenologists had them in their consulting rooms and enthusiastic amateurs bought them as mantelpiece decorations.

In 1886 Lorenzo founded the British Phrenological Society, which flourished well into the twentieth century. Amazingly, it only became defunct in 1967.

THE PRINCIPLES OF PHRENOLOGY

The phrenologists claimed that phrenology was a science or system of mental philosophy founded upon the physiology of the brain. The fundamental principle was that the brain is the organ of the mind and that it is composed of a number of smaller organs which they called faculties, each of which governs a function of the mind or of personality. They believed that there were four main divisions.

The front portion of the head was said to be associated with intellectual functions, where the thinking, planning and organising, reasoning and intuitional faculties were located.

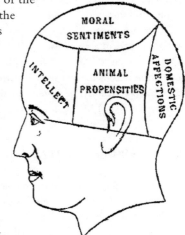

The four phrenological divisions.

The back of the head was associated with the domestic or social faculties, to do with love of home and family, of children, animals and friends. They described some of these in delightfully arcane language, such as the very first three faculties located at the back of the head:

amativeness (love and attraction towards the opposite sex, libido)
conjugality (faithfulness towards one's partner)
philoprogenitiveness (love of children, animals and pets)

The sides of the head were associated with the animal propensities. These were the self-preserving faculties of courage, economy, cautiousness, prudence, hunger, and so on.

The top of the head indicated the moral and religious faculties, not surprisingly, since these would be rated above all else by the Victorians and would be expected to be the ones nearest to heaven and God.

Gall had delineated twenty-six faculties, but gradually the number swelled to forty-six.

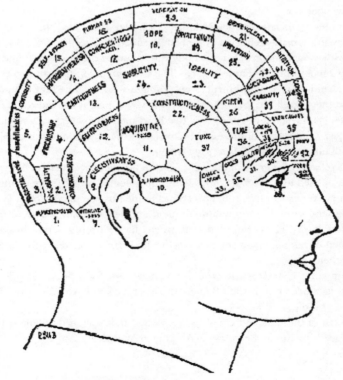

The phrenological faculties.

QUESTIONABLE RESEARCH

According to phrenological principles, anyone who was touched by genius in some sphere of endeavour should have an obviously developed part of their skull, which would correspond with the part of the brain that gave them their genius. In order to ascertain this, for it would be an important piece of evidence in support of their theories, phrenologists took whatever opportunities they could to examine the heads of living geniuses. In some cases they also tried to examine the skulls of those who had recently departed.

In 1809 the celebrated composer Joseph Haydn (1732–1809) died and was buried in Vienna. Austria was at that time at war with Napoleon and the interment of the composer was only regarded as a temporary measure. Shortly after the burial two men bribed the sextant and then dug the grave and severed the head. The two men were Joseph Carl Rosenbaum, the secretary of Haydn's former employers, and Johan Nepomuk Peter, a prison governor. They both had an interest in phrenology and were eager to find the seat of Haydn's genius. They prepared the head and examined it, recording that the musical faculty bump was inordinately large, as would be expected. Reverentially, the skull was kept in a black wooden box.

Some ten years later, Prince Nikolaus Esterhazy II recalled that he had not had Haydn's remains reburied as he had intended and arranged for this to be done with some honour. When the body was exhumed the head was found to be missing and a justifiable furore erupted. The two phrenologists managed to hide the head and escaped punishment, even although at a later time they did provide a replacement skull! The real head was kept in secret, first by Rosenbaum's family and then Peter's. It was not until 1954 that head and body were finally reunited.

In 1827 a similar but unsuccessful bid was made by phrenologists to obtain the head of Ludwig van Beethoven (1770–1827).

In 1834, when the grave of the great Scottish poet Robert Burns of Ayr (1759–96) was opened to make way for his wife, phrenologists took the opportunity to make a plaster cast of his skull. This was examined by the phrenologist George Combe who wrote a monograph about it entitled *Phrenological Development of Robert Burns*. He concluded that Burns had a highly active brain and enhanced development of the faculties of the brain associated with language and mathematics.

The former characteristic would have been apt for a poet, yet the latter is dubious, since all of his life Robert Burns proved to have little aptitude for business or money.

The cast of the skull and Combe's report are on display in the Robert Burns Birthplace Museum in the village of Alloway in Ayrshire.

PHRENOLOGY IN PRACTICE

Visiting a phrenologist was rather like attending a doctor. Most phrenologists had example charts, casts of skulls and brains about their consulting rooms, which they would use to explain the nature of their craft. They would take a history, absorbing what information the client wished to give to them, and then they would examine the head with callipers, tape measures and various other ingenious measuring gadgets to build up a picture of the contours of the person's skull. This could then be translated into a detailed analysis of the person's head, ending in the phrenologist's opinion of their potential, or otherwise, for various endeavours.

A particularly popular part of their practice was assessing couples for compatibility. How successful they were is hard to determine, since divorce was not common. On that basis, they may well have been able to demonstrate excellent results.

PHRENO-MESMERISM

Simply analysing someone's potential would not be considered enough, of course. People would want the phrenologist to be able to do something in order to increase their potential, and perhaps to reduce any faculty that the person thought was not desirable. The question was, how could you do that? The answer was to be found in that other great science or art that had enjoyed such a vogue – mesmerism.

Dr Joseph Rhodes Buchanan (1814–99) was a professor of medicine and physiology at the Eclectic Medical Institute in Covington, Kentucky in the USA. He was a confirmed phrenologist and was intensely interested in mesmerism. From his physiology background he believed that experimentation was important to advance science, and he believed that mesmerism provided an excellent tool to investigate the principles of phrenology. Accordingly, he began studying the effects of stroking the prominences on people's heads when they were in a mesmeric or hypnotic trance. He was convinced that by doing so he could enhance the faculty associated with that particular bump. In 1842 he coined the term 'phreno-mesmerism' for this new development.

In 1843 he produced his own phrenological map, which he believed gave insight into some of the more mysterious or occult senses of man. In particular he discovered an area that he equated with the faculty of 'sensibility'. This he believed to be associated with psychic senses, such as the ability to derive information about a person by handling an object that once belonged to them. This ability he called 'psychometry', or soul-reading. It would be an ability that many mediums would later claim to have, or that they would be able to tap into by contacting the spirit world.

Many phrenologists took up the practice of hypnosis, which is not difficult to learn, and make it known that they were trained in both phrenology and mesmerism and that they could solve all manner of problems with phreno-mesmerism. Essentially, under a hypnotic trance they would massage areas of the skull and give hypnotic suggestions and post-hypnotic suggestions that the relevant faculty would be enhanced. There is no doubt that with hypnotisable people (and probably 95 per cent of people can be hypnotised to a greater or lesser extent) this would have achieved good results. The practitioner would probably establish a good reputation.

One such phrenologist was Spencer Timothy Hall (1812–85) who began his career as a printer. Possibly as a result of publishing work on phrenology he became intensely interested in the subject and undertook training. He was the first secretary of the Sheffield Phrenological Society and later became an honorary member of the Phrenological Society of Glasgow.

In 1841 he took up the practice of mesmerism and in 1843 founded The Phreno-Magnet, or Mirror of Nature. Among his celebrated clients was the famous writer Harriet Martineau, whom he treated with phreno-mesmerism.

Another was Dr James George Davey (1813–85) who was for a time colonial secretary to Ceylon, 'responsible for the care of the insane'. He did much work with both phrenology and phreno-mesmerism and found it to be the most effective method of treatment that he had at his disposal. It has to be remembered that conventional medicine had virtually nothing else to offer other than various types of physical restraint, cold baths, plunges or the powerful opiate drug laudanum.

He later returned to England and held posts as medical superintendent of several asylums and attained high office in various medical societies. His written works were highly regarded and his status as a qualified doctor did much to keep phreno-mesmerism at the forefront of medical practice during the Victorian era, at least until phrenology began to decline in popularity.

SUPPORT IN HIGH PLACES

Although it had many detractors, phrenology also had powerful friends. There were eminent professors of anatomy, surgeons, doctors, lawyers and clergymen who professed an interest and a belief that it was a subject that held profound truth. It seemed so logical, and since it had been backed up by anatomical dissection and could be shown by the use of prepared specimens and charts to have an almost tangible basis, it seemed perfectly plausible. It fitted neatly into the scientific world, somewhere between anatomy and anthropology, and it promised to unlock the mysteries of the mind.

One of its most ardent supporters was Professor Alfred Russel Wallace (1823–1913), explorer, geographer, naturalist and biologist who, independently from Darwin, came up with a similar theory of evolution. Indeed, there are many who would claim that his name should be held in as high esteem as that of Charles Darwin, who published his theory before he had originally intended to ensure that the world knew about his theory before Wallace's.

Wallace said: 'The phrenologist has shown that he is able to read character like an open book, and to lay bare the hidden springs of conduct with an accuracy that the most intimate friends cannot approach.' We shall hear more of Wallace in Part Two: Mediums.

The American Professor Elmer Gates (1859–1923) was another famous Victorian-era scientist. He invented the foam fire extinguisher, an air-conditioning system and an improved electric iron. He was also extremely interested in psychology, the study of which occupied much of his time. He wrote: 'It is a sound scientific basis for character reading. Under the usual methods of education, children develop less than one tenth of their brain cells, but by wise guidance those fallow areas may be made more active.'

THE END OF PHRENOLOGY

Phrenology was never completely accepted, even in its heyday in the middle of the nineteenth century. It had always had its critics, who could be every bit as vociferous as its supporters. Undoubtedly one of the problems was the fact that anyone could practice, the result being that a great many charlatans did jump on the bandwagon. In the tradition of the mountebank they would appear at fairs, at markets and in the music halls, offering exactly what people wanted. They fed egos, lied blatantly and probably went on to other forms of chicanery when a more profitable line came along. On the other hand, it is probable that a great many people did truly believe in what they were doing and managed to delude themselves into thinking that they were reading character from the shape of the head, rather than intuitively judging character by observation and absorbing what the client was telling them.

Gradually, though, medical science started to discredit phrenology. The discipline of neurology was being developed and it became clear that the brain was not made up of such faculties as the phrenologists proposed. Nor did the bumps and prominences on the skull reflect the shape of the brain underneath.

Although it started to lose credibility in the latter quarter of the Victorian era, it did not give up the ghost until well into the twentieth century. Despite medical science it still seemed credible to many people, in the same way that people still find palm-reading or any other predictive art plausible.

THE ICON LIVES ON

The phrenological chart and the busts that were so ubiquitous in Victorian times are still all around. They have attained iconic status, not for phrenology but as an image of the mind. Psychology textbooks, popular self-help books, websites and all manner of adverts still use that phrenological head. The practitioners have come and gone, the mountains of books that they wrote are no longer read, and their philosophy has been derided and jettisoned to the footnotes of history, yet the iconic image persists. It does so, I think, because the whole thing did seem so plausible.

AND FINALLY

The great and good having once spoken in favour of it were ever after accepted as advocates. 'I never knew I had an inventive talent until phrenology told me so. I was a stranger to myself until then.' So said the great inventor Thomas Alva Edison (1847–1931). Perhaps we do have something to thank phrenology for.

6

DENTAL MEDDLERS

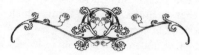

There was never yet philosopher
That could endure the toothache patiently.

Much Ado About Nothing
William Shakespeare (1564–1616)

Teeth have always been of prime concern to people. The pain of toothache, the agony of gumboils, the smell of halitosis, and the unpleasant appearance of black, yellow or dirty teeth have caused people to seek the ministrations of all manner of practitioner over the centuries.

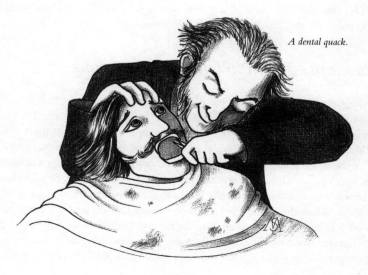

A dental quack.

THE TOOTHWORM AND URINE GARGLES

The ancients believed that tooth decay was the result of a toothworm that got inside the tooth and ate it away. The Babylonians attempted to smoke these irritating creatures out by a quite ingenious method. As long ago as 2250 BC they mixed henbane with beeswax and then heated it in order to produce smoke. This smoke was directed into the carious hole, after which the hole was filled with a sort of gum mastic and more henbane.

The Egyptians had specialist physicians who would deal with teeth and gum problems. They seemed to do little in the way of removal, their treatments mainly consisting of magic rituals, charms and sacrifices to appease the gods, then the use of various purgative enemas and masticatory agents which when chewed would encourage the production of saliva.

The Etruscans in the first millennium BC seem to have been the first people to use false teeth. They even made bridges so that false teeth could be anchored to normal teeth by rings of gold. Archaeologists are unsure, however, whether these were designed for the use of the living, or whether they were made to enhance the look of the body after death.

The Greeks actually recognised that sometimes teeth need to be pulled in order to allow an abscess to be released. The great Hippocrates even invented some crude forceps for the purpose.

The Romans built on the work of the Greeks and developed a series of instruments specifically for work on the teeth. They also worked gold into crowns for the teeth and different types of forceps for tooth-pulling. Mostly dental care was restricted to the nobility and caries, gum disease and, ultimately, toothlessness were the norms for the bulk of the population.

As for mouthwashes, one of the most widely advocated in Roman times was urine, especially the freshly passed urine of young boys.

THE MIDDLE AGES AND THE TOOTH-PULLERS

Although universities were starting to spring up across Europe, at Padua, Salerno, Bologna, Montpellier and Paris, and in Britain at Oxford and Cambridge, knowledge about teeth and their care did not really advance from the days of the Romans. Medical texts were reprinted, but the treatments and recommendations were still a mix of magic and multi-ingredient medication, coupled with purgation and emesis.

St Apollonia of Alexandria was the patron saint of toothaches. She had been a deaconess who was martyred by the Romans in AD 249, after riots inspired by her teachings. When she refused to renounce her religion she had her teeth pulled one by one and her jaw broken. She then threw herself into a fire after saying in her prayer that she hoped no one would experience her pain and suffering or the agony of toothache. Such was the power of the Church and the belief in the saint that many would probably receive relief from toothache by praying to her. Whether that relief was the result of saintly intervention or the power of the placebo effect is another question.

For the common people recourse was often made to remedies from the old 'leech' books (from the Anglo-Saxon *leche*, meaning 'leach', the sign of a doctor). These would advise that caries could be cleared of our old friend the toothworm, by the smoke of henbane, or after being packed with mixtures containing substances like ground beetles, lizards and raven dung.

Of course tooth-pulling would be the most effective way of dealing with agonising toothache. Putting up with the pain of the extraction would for many be preferable to the agony of the underlying abscess or nerve pain. Physicians did not generally like to get their hands dirty, so tooth-pulling was done by barber-surgeons or itinerant tooth-pullers.

These travelling tooth-pullers or mountebanks could make a decent living by going from town to town and market to market, setting up their stall with a flag or poster of St Apollonia, a string of wooden teeth or a carved crocodile with sharp teeth. They would climb on their crude box or stage and bring in crowds with their claims of being able to pull teeth without pain, or with such speed that there would be minimal pain. Any teeth that proved difficult to extract would be left alone with the advice that they must not be removed, since the pain they had experienced was because they were 'eye teeth'. This was of course another of the myths that was promulgated, that they were in some way connected to the eyes and that blindness could result if they were pulled.

The favoured instrument was called 'The Pelican', a large instrument like pliers, which would inspire fear in the mind of the sufferer as a tooth-puller advanced with it poised.

The tooth-pullers also offered quack remedies such as mouth washes that were guaranteed to whiten black teeth and turn them into ivory. Doubtless they had many tricks and ploys up their sleeves or in the mouths of the paid confederates in the audience. By all accounts these mountebanks were great crowd drawers with their teeth-pulling, for such is the darker side of human nature that people often revel in watching the misfortune of others.

A ROYAL DENTIST

King James IV (1473–1513) was an interesting monarch. He came to the throne at the age of 15 and proved himself to be a one of the most remarkable of men by anyone's standards. He brought peace to Scotland by ensuring a treaty with King Henry VII. He then concentrated on his own people, believing that to rule effectively the ruling classes should be educated. He therefore decreed that all landowning families should send their sons to school and then on to one of the three ancient universities of St Andrews, Glasgow or Aberdeen.

He himself was interested in the healing arts and actually practiced both surgery and dentistry. Indeed, there are documents in the Surgeon's Hall Museum in Edinburgh, which is the official museum of the Royal College of Surgeons of Edinburgh, which show that he received fees for pulling teeth. He firmly believed that there should be some sort of regulation of both dentistry and surgery. Accordingly, he granted a royal seal to the barber-surgeons of Edinburgh in 1506. This Seal of Cause (or charter of principles) stated that:

> ... that no manner of person occupy or practise any points of our said craft of surgery... unless he be worthy and expert in all points belonging to the said craft, diligently and expertly examined and admitted by the Maisters of the said craft and that he know Anatomy and the nature and complexion of every member of the human body... for every man ocht to know the nature and substance of everything that he works or else he is negligent.

OUT OF THE DARKNESS

As we saw in Chapter 2, the Georgian era was the Golden Age of Quackery. One truly spectacular dental meddler who became quite famous in the 1770s was the mountebank Martin van Butchall, who rode about London on a large white horse painted with purple spots. He carried a bone before him and declared that he could draw teeth painlessly and also manufacture a set of false teeth and fit them absolutely painlessly.

A natural showman, he went beyond the bounds of taste and introduced a macabre reason why clients should go to see him, which they did in droves. When his first wife died he had her embalmed; had glass eyes fitted to the corpse and kept her in a glass case in his hall. There he introduced her to all of his guests.

His second wife was not so enamoured by the presence of his first wife in the family home, so van Butchell reluctantly donated the body to the Royal College of Surgeons, where it was kept until it was destroyed along with many other exhibits when the building was bombed during the Second World War.

Pierre Fauchard (1678–1761) is regarded as the father of modern dentistry. His landmark book *Le Chirurgien Dentiste* (*The Surgeon Dentist*) was first published in 1728 and set the standard for the emerging discipline as a specific specialty of surgery. Drawing on his early experience as a ship's surgeon, he wrote about surgical procedures to treat diseased gums and teeth and all manner of injuries to the mouth and jaws. He used silk, linen and metal suture material and taught how to make dentures, bridges and crowns.

He also advocated the use of the toothbrush. It was only at the end of the seventeenth century that people began to use them with any regularity.

Fauchard's work found its way across the channel and in the 1750s the word 'dentist' was adopted into English. An apprenticeship type of profession arose, it taking four or five years to become experienced enough to set up a sign or a brass plate and establish a practice of one's own.

WATERLOO TEETH

The craft of dentistry began to develop. Interestingly, as trade increased so too did the importation of sugar from abroad. Many people developed a sweet tooth, which ultimately was followed by rotting teeth. Cause and effect was not yet apparent, and although surgical dentistry was improving many dentists still believed in the mythical toothworm. Their main function was to pull teeth and prepare false ones.

The best false teeth that could be obtained, however, were human ones. Although dentists had experimented with porcelain, ivory and bone, none of these materials was ever as good as the enamel-covered human tooth. This created a huge problem, of course, since they were hard to come by and the law of supply and demand forced the price of dentures ever upward. Some dentists advertised to buy teeth from people willing to sell theirs for a guinea or two a tooth, the highest price going for the incisors.

George Washington, the first president of the United States under the Constitution, was reputed to have a wooden set of dentures. In fact this is a myth, since he had a very fine set of dentures consisting of a smoothed plate of hippopotamus ivory into which human, horse and pig teeth were inserted.

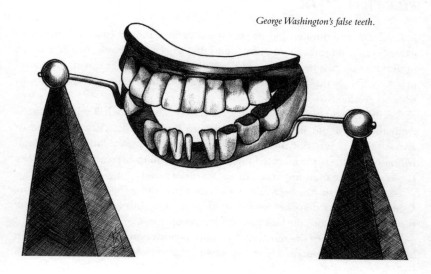

George Washington's false teeth.

The Battle of Waterloo in 1815 resulted in a new phenomenon; the wholesale removal of teeth from the slain. Over 50,000 men died and there was a rich harvest of teeth made by persons unknown. These were sold to dentists and the term 'Waterloo teeth' was coined. Although dentists would deny that the teeth they used came from the battle, the name stuck for decades afterwards and it was suspected that many dentures owed some of their teeth to the young, fit and healthy men who had fallen at Waterloo.

THE RESURRECTIONISTS

In the years following Waterloo, right up until the Anatomy Act of 1832, body-snatching was rife. Cemeteries were full to capacity in many of the cities, many churchyards having had to bury bodies one on top of each other. As a result, early in Queen Victoria's reign larger cemeteries were established, such as the ring of seven great cemeteries around London – Highgate, Abney Green, Brompton, Kensal Green, Nunhead, West Norwood and Tower Hamlets.

Body-snatching was a lucrative, but dangerous occupation, for it played on people's fears. The desecration of the grave, the removal of loved ones and the mutilation of their bodies filled the public with horror. Despite the risk of transportation to the colonies or execution if caught, grave-robbers could make a substantial living. The trade in Waterloo teeth also meant that dentists as well as doctors might pay handsomely for teeth if the bodies had decayed past their usefulness to the anatomists.

FILL THAT CAVITY

Many dental practitioners did attempt to fill cavities. Indeed Fauchard advocated using tin or gold foil, although he found that tin was more effective. It was not until the 1830s that dentists started to prepare the cavity by removing the caries first. Accordingly they started using a burr and thimble to remove as much carious tissue as possible.

A drill based on the Archimedean screw; essentially a hand drill was introduced from the 1840s, but it had to be used with both hands as it was limited in accessibility. It was not until 1871 when the American dentist James Beall Morrison (1829–1919) invented the foot treadle drill to overcome this problem. It was one of the most important dental inventions ever.

The dental chair had been another advance that almost became a dental icon. Custom-made wooden ones were introduced in 1850 with special curves to allow the patient to get into the best position for the operator.

In the early part of the nineteenth century dentists started experimenting with amalgams as filling agents. Generally, however, gold was preferred, and although silver-mercury amalgams called *succedaneum*, meaning 'artificial substitute', were introduced, it did not become used generally until towards the close of the century. Indeed, in America its use was banned and a dentist could be struck off their register for using it.

VICTORIAN DENTAL MEDDLERS

The middle of the century really marks the period when dentistry started to come of age. Rather like medicine it was unregulated. The Medical Act of 1858 saw the introduction of the General Medical Council and the General Medical Register, requiring all doctors to hold qualifying certificates, diplomas or degrees. The equivalent General Dental Council was not established until 1956, almost a century later. So there was still room for dental meddling.

Dental meddlers still practiced in the same manner than they had done back in the Middle Ages, by visiting towns and markets and setting up temporary shows or premises and whipping out teeth. Pain relief was always the big problem, but in the 1830s and 1840s there was a resurgence of interest in mesmerism.

The man who brought this about was an English surgeon called John Elliotson. While he was in France he saw a demonstration of mesmerism and soon found that it was not difficult to mesmerise a patient. He even found that with adequate preparation he could perform operations on people while they were in a trance.

Next, John Esdaile, a Scottish surgeon working in India, took up the practice of mesmerism and performed numerous tricky operations using only mesmerism. He believed that the phenomenon worked rather as Mesmer had suggested the century before, through the passage of a sort of healing fluid. This was disputed by another Scottish doctor, James Braid, who coined the term 'neuro-hypnotism', for the state that was induced. In time it became shortened to 'hypnosis'.

News about this wonderful phenomenon and its potential spread around the empire and soon many 'professional' mesmerists were performing around the country. Some actually used it to extract teeth painlessly and so had truly crossed into the realm of dental meddlers. It seemed that a great power had been unlocked and for a while it seemed that nothing could equal it.

Then, in 1846 in America, Dr William T.G. Morton (1819–68) introduced ether to permit painless extractions. From then mesmerism as a dental aid seemed to decline and anyone who could get access to ether could potentially remove teeth relatively painlessly, without all the seeming dramatics of mesmerism. People who were not dentists could therefore get in on the act, including medical students, doctors, herbalists and pharmacists.

REGULATION AND THE END OF DENTAL MEDDLING BEGINS

It is important to appreciate, of course, that not everyone involved in dentistry in Victorian times was a meddler. There would have been a great many practitioners who were remarkably skilful and who could perform extractions, fill cavities and treat abscesses perfectly well. Indeed, some of these reputable dentists railed against the quacks and meddlers who purported to have skill that they did not possess, and who did far more to harm than to help.

In a letter to *The Lancet* in 1855 a young Croydon dentist by the name of Samuel Lee Rymer suggested that there was a need to form a college of dental surgery. Following the letter he called a public meeting to establish a dental society and introduce professional dental examinations for dental surgeons. In 1856 the College of Dentists of England was formed. There was initial rivalry from the Royal College of Surgeons who felt that all surgeons, dental or not, should be qualified surgeons. This seemed to have the effect of other small organisations of dentists forming in other cities of the country. After much internal politics the Dentists' Act was passed in 1878.

This stated that:

> From and after 1st August 1879 a person shall not be entitled to take or use the name
> of dentist or dental practitioner, or any other name, title or addition or description
> implying that he is registered under this act, or that he is a person specially qualified
> to practice dentistry unless he is registered under the Act.

Doctors were still permitted to practice dentistry, and as long as they did not administer anaesthetics, pharmacists could also extract teeth.

This was not quite the end of dental meddling, but it was the beginning of the end. People began to realise that it paid to ensure that the person treating them was properly qualified. If he wasn't then you were simply putting your teeth in their hands, for good or ill. For people who could not afford proper treatment then tooth extraction might have been all that they wanted, for once the tooth was gone the problem was gone.

7

SNAKE OIL, HAIR TONICS AND CARBOLIC SMOKE

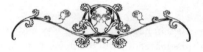

We saw in Chapter 2, The Golden Age of Quackery, that from the seventeenth century doctors and medical meddlers were manufacturing their own medicines. There was no obligation to list the ingredients. Indeed, most people wanted to keep that secret to prevent others from attempting to cash in on their panacea. Some, like Ward's Pill and Drop, contained active or even highly toxic ingredients, which they wanted to disguise. While others, mainly medical meddlers with no actual medical or pharmaceutical credentials, would wish to conceal the fact that their remedies contained nothing useful whatever.

PATENT MEDICINES AND SNAKE OIL

The term 'patent medicine' originated in a 'patent of royal favour', which was granted to those who supplied medicines to the royal family. Later it referred to an official government protection, which would give the owner of the patent exclusivity of manufacture. However, this was often flouted and was almost impossible to enforce. The result was that many people simply started manufacturing potions, pills and embrocations of all sorts, labelling and selling them through whatever outlets they could. Patent medicine sellers could be found at fairs, markets, theatres or with strolling player groups. And of course, it was the ideal product for the mountebank medical meddler; any self-respecting meddler would have his own product to peddle.

In America snake oil was regarded in the same derogatory light. In fact, snake oil is a traditional Chinese medicine of great antiquity, used as an embrocation to rub on painful parts of the body. It is prepared from the Chinese water snake (*Enhydris chinensis*) and used for all manner of rheumatic and arthritic pain by practitioners. It found its way to America during the time of railroad expansion and was brought by Chinese workers. Along with many such rubefacients[3] it may have helped, which would account for many medicine shows selling it widely. The thing is that it was then usually done with great gusto about its qualities. A good medicine showman would probably extend the list of conditions that any preparation could be used for, the result being that most of these things were ultimately sold as panaceas to cure everything from piles to baldness, and from minor illnesses to the most serious. The dangers of such salesmanship are all too obvious.

DAFFY'S ELIXIR

This was a very popular patent medicine that was widely sold in Britain and the United States in the eighteenth and nineteenth centuries. It was originally marketed as stomach cramp medicine that became extended for use in all stomach conditions and, ultimately, was advocated by peddlers as a panacea that would help anything, including epilepsy, dropsy, scurvy and gout.

It is thought to have been invented by the Reverend Thomas Daffy, the rector of Redmile in Leicestershire in 1647.

DR JOHN HOOPER'S FEMALE PILLS

These were pills advocated to help women if afflicted with 'hysteria', which was regarded as a female complaint for centuries. Hippocrates had suggested back in the fifth century BC that it was caused by a wandering womb. Indeed, the word comes from the Greek *hystera*, meaning 'uterus' or 'womb'.

In 1743 Dr John Hooper patented these pills as a means of treating all period problems and difficulties that young women might be susceptible to. Indeed, it was advertised as: 'The best medicine ever discovered for young women, when afflicted with what is commonly called the irregularities.'

He said the pills were: '... also excellent for the palpitations of the heart, giddiness, loathing of food ... a dejected countenance, a dislike to exercise and conversation, and likewise for the scurvy.' It was also advised after childbirth and during the menopause, but not during pregnancy. This led many women to think that it could induce unwanted pregnancies.

....

3. A rubefacient is a preparation that is applied to the skin and rubbed on. It will produce some skin irritation which may over-ride the pain from the underlying tissues.

JACKSON'S TINCTURE

This was a remedy advertised in the *Cumberland Pacquet* of Tuesday 22 April 1777. It survived well into the nineteenth century:

> for the Rheumatism, Gravel, Stone, Cholic, or Griping of the Bowels, or any such like windy disorders; it not only gives perfect ease, but if continued taking, one bottle or two will entirely remove and destroy the cause; and is infallible in disorders of the fair sex, either young or old (it is superior to any medicine extant). Likewise burns, scalds, bruises, strains, old ulcers, or swellings of any kind, especially white swellings, it cures to admiration. Price 1s. the bottle.

BOTT'S NEW INVENTED CORN-SALVE

The qualities of this corn plaster seemed to extend well beyond its original intention of helping sore feet:

> THIS SALVE is the most effectual remedy for Corns ever yet invented, taking them entirely away, though of ever so long standing, the method of using it is quite safe and gives no pain; neither does it occasion any inconveniency during the time of cure. It is likewise an effectual remedy for Warts, washing them away unperceivably, without making any kind of sore or scar, let them be of ever so long standing. It also cures strains and bruises, and takes down hard swellings, though ever so bad, in a short time, dispersing the congealed blood that settles in them, and soon effects a cure; by applying a fresh plaister once a week. But be sure you don't apply it to green wounds, or where the skin is broke, for there it will not be serviceable. It will keep its virtues for seven years, by sea or land, if occasion require it; keep it a distance from the fire, but dry … Price One Shilling the box.

VANDOUR'S NERVOUS PILLS

Remedies for all manner of nervous disorder were also sought after – and provided. Vandour's nervous pills were widely used:

> SO UNIVERSALLY esteemed for their good effects in all nervous disorders, lowness of spirits, headaches, tremblings, vain fears, and wanderings of the mind, frightful dreams, catchings, startings, anxieties, dimness, with the appearance of specks before the eyes, loss of memory, cholics, cramps, convulsions, hysteric fits, hypochondriac complaints, and the falling sickness.

They prevent sickness at the stomach, and take off that sense of fullness after meals, and that swelling of the flesh in damp weather, which so greatly affect persons of relaxed fibres; they give a serene cheerfulness of disposition, in the place of those horrors, which so dreadfully oppress people of weak nerves. Price Two Shillings and Six-pence the box, which contains fifty pills.

ALLAN'S ANTI-FAT PILLS

This was an American patent medicine widely used in the nineteenth century from the 1870s onwards. It was a concoction of marine lichen, which would have been full of iodides. These could have an effect on the thyroid gland and they were said to prevent the body from converting food into fat.

DR GREY'S ELECTRIC FAT REDUCING PILLS

Not to be outdone, these British pills were advertised in the *Illustrated Sporting and Drama News* of 1893. They were said to be effective in 'rapidly and quite safely dissolving superfluous fat, permanently curing corpulency, and improving the general health and figure'.

THE AMMONIAPHONE

This was a quite interesting gadget, consisting of a silver tube filled with chemicals and aromatic oils. Its inventor, Dr Carter Moffat, believed that the southern Italian plains provided a perfect healing atmosphere. He tried to simulate the air, which he had analysed and found to be rich in ammonia and hydrogen peroxide.

He advocated it for the treatment of throat and chest diseases such as asthma, bronchitis, consumption, coughs, colds, loss of voice and deafness. He also marketed it as a voice tone improver.

It sold widely from the 1870s until the end of the century. The user breathed in through the centre of the tube. Its advert claimed that it was used by many of the famous people of the day.

REGULATION NEEDED

The fact that patent remedies could be produced and sold without revealing all their ingredients was open to all sorts of abuse and was incredibly dangerous. Eventually, certain drugs like alcohol and opiate drugs like cocaine and opium had to be indicated on the labels. However, that was as far as it went. As long as they were labelled they could be sold. The quantities were quite another matter. Accordingly, people who wished to partake in strong drugs could do so by buying certain patent medicines. It was extremely dangerous and accidental overdoses could easily be taken by young and old. There was need for legislation.

The extravagant claims also needed to be addressed, as some of the advertisements we have looked at have exemplified.

THE CARBOLIC SMOKE BOMB COMPANY

One of the most significant cases in English law is that of Carlill vs. The Carbolic Smoke Bomb Company. It came about because the company manufactured a device that created a carbolic smoke ball. This, they claimed, would prevent influenza. They went further than that. In 1892 they offered a £100 reward to anyone who used the smoke ball and went on to contract influenza. Mrs Carlill used it and got influenza then claimed her £100. The company referred her to their lawyers, saying that she was impertinent in her demand and that the advertisement was merely advertising 'puff' and not seriously meant to be a contract. On her part she argued that they had made an offer, which she had accepted.

Mrs Carlill successfully sued them and the rules of 'offer' and 'acceptance' were then established as a precedent in English contract law.

MIXER'S CANCER & SCROFULA SYRUP

This was an American patent remedy that was said to cure cancer! It was made from various roots and alcohol and was sold widely in the 1880s and 1890s.

In 1906 the Pure Food and Drug Act was passed. Almost overnight it put a stop to the manufacture of dangerous and poisonous patent medicines in the United States. In 1909, the purveyor, Charles Mixer of Hastings, Michigan, who was operating as Dr Mixer, had a judgement made against him under the Pure Food and Drug Act that he was misrepresenting a drug. His claims were extravagant and 'patently' untrue!

PART TWO

MEDIUMS

8

THE COMING OF SPIRITUALISM

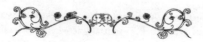

For who can wonder that man should feel a vague belief in tales of disembodied spirits wandering through those places which they once dearly affected, when he himself, scarcely less separated from his old world than they, is for ever lingering upon past emotions and bygone times, and hovering, the ghost of his former self, about the places and people that warmed his heart of old?

Master Humphrey's Clock
Charles Dickens

Most religions believe in the survival of the spirit in some form. Spiritualism, which really came into being during the Victorian era, went further than that. It stated that not only did the spirit survive, but that the spirits of the dead can and do communicate with the living. It was also purported that not everyone had the ability to communicate with the disembodied spirits, but people with a particular gift could do so on their behalf. Such individuals were termed mediums.

As we saw in Chapter 2 The Golden Age of Quackery, there were people such as the Count of Cagliostro who professed to have special powers and the gift to communicate with the dead. The practice of necromancy was of course a dangerous practice in those days, as Cagliostro himself found out. To claim that one could communicate with the spirits was considered heresy, the punishment for which could be terrible.

Things were changing in the nineteenth century and there was a much more open and curious attitude. The scientific discoveries in physics and chemistry had shown that there were ways of tapping into energies that had not been apparent before. Engineers and inventors were creating new machines, new techniques and new ways of doing things that were transforming lives. There was a general belief that there was a whole new world of possibilities, a range of energies that existed but which had always been unseen. There was no reason, therefore, why experimenters in other areas of life should not also discover wonderful things. And what could be more wonderful than to be able to demonstrate that the spirit did survive death? The time was ripe; the era of credulity had come about. It just needed someone to make that first communication and demonstrate that there was life eternal and that one's loved ones were waiting somewhere close by in a spirit world to send their messages back.

THE FOX SISTERS

The story of spiritualism as a movement and quasi-religion starts in America in 1848 with the Fox family of New York. Essentially it began with all the ingredients that are needed for a good ghost story: a creepy old house, a bad and grisly reputation about it and stories of a ghost and strange noises and bumps in the night.

It was to such a house that the Fox family moved into on 11 December 1847. There were three sisters in the family, Leah (1814–90), Margaret (1833–93) and Kate (1837–92). They also had an older brother called David who had left home. Leah, being older, was already married and living in Rochester as Mrs Fish. Although they did not realise it the two younger sisters would soon find themselves at the forefront of an amazing phenomenon that would sweep America and then travel across the Atlantic to Britain.

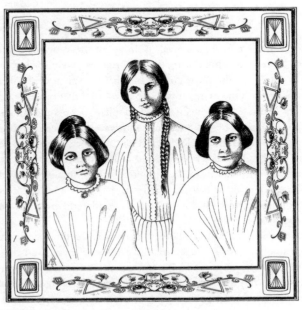

The Fox sisters.

It has to be said that there are several different accounts of what happened to the sisters. Inevitably, considering the nature of the events and their bearing upon the birth of spiritualism, there is great controversy surrounding the whole story. Let us first of all look at things as they seemed to unfold.

The Fox family lived quite contentedly in the house until spring 1848 when they became aware of strange noises. These took the form of knocks and raps as if furniture was being moved. These became more and more frequent until one night they seemed to go on unabated for several hours. The parents searched the house but could find no cause. Yet the noises continued and Kate, the youngest child, discovered that she could actually communicate with whatever was causing the noises by rapping on furniture herself. She found that she could ask questions and demonstrated by snapping her fingers. She established that a question could be answered by one rap for 'yes' and two for 'no'.

Her mother, Mrs Fox, then began asking questions, receiving the same affirmative or negative responses. Soon it was established that the replier did not belong to the living world, but that it was a spirit. More than that, she found out that the spirit was of a peddler who had been murdered and that his spirit was restless and unhappy. Not content with just investigating matters themselves, Mr and Mrs Fox asked the spirit if it would mind also communicating with their neighbours. This it agreed to, with similar results.

This occasioned a search in the cellar and a plan to dig up the floor. Initial attempts had to be stopped because the hole filled up with water. When the summer came and the water had dried up they were able to resume. At a depth of 5ft they found evidence of quicklime, hair and bones. A medical opinion stated that these were human remains.

There was an inevitable stir caused in the newspapers. The attention that it caused to the family was not welcomed by the parents who were concerned for the girls, so they decided to send them away for a while. Kate was sent to stay with her brother, David, and Margaret was sent to her elder sister, Leah Fish, in Rochester. The strange rapping noises seemed to follow both girls.

A friend, Isaac Post, and his wife, both staunch Quakers and advocates of temperance, abolition of slavery and the rights of women, invited the girls to their home. There the phenomenon was demonstrated and the Posts convinced them that they had a God-given gift, and that the messages they were able to give as a result should be shared with the world.

This background is interesting, because the surge of interest at first came from the Quaker community and among people who were like-minded. Honest, sober, hard-working folk who were liberal in their outlook and desirous of equality for all. As such they may have been overly credulous, but significantly they would be perceived as being strictly honest and devoid of guile or intention to deceive.

The Fox sisters became a phenomenon. It is said that Leah Fish took matters in hand and began to seriously promote the two younger girls as mediums. Within a short period of time they had become famous around New York and attracted the great and the good, including luminaries like the novelist James Fenimore Cooper, the poet and editor of the *New York Evening Post* William Cullen Bryant, and the journalist and abolitionist William Lloyd Garrison. It was not long before they were making the considerable sum of $150 a night. At meetings there would always be mention of the need to support the good causes of temperance, abolition and women's suffrage with which they were linked.

At séances, the spirits communicated by raps, table turning and spirit writing. We shall consider some of these phenomena later.

Ironically, both of the young sisters found the attention hard to deal with and despite their temperance background they both began drinking wine. It is said that in later life they both became addicted to alcohol and their deaths may have been drink-related.

The touch paper had been lit, however, and spiritualism flourished. Many other mediums surfaced and started to give séances across the country. Some, as we shall find out in a moment, became famous and crossed the Atlantic to bring the word to Britain, where it was quickly taken up.

Marriage eventually separated the sisters. Leah's husband died and she married a Wall Street banker. Margaret married the naval medical officer and arctic explorer Dr Elisha Kane. At that point Margaret gave up her spiritualism and converted to Catholicism, which she practiced until her husband died in 1857.

Kate continued her good work and became ever more famous and sought after by the rich, powerful and bereaved. In 1861 she was engaged exclusively by the wealthy banker Charles F. Livermore, whose wife Estelle had recently passed away. Over the following five years she gave him some 400 private readings. The phenomena that she produced, apparently under stringent conditions, with witnesses present (and that included working in a locked room and with both hands held), was amazing. Lights, ectoplasm and spirit writing were produced. Images of Estelle appeared and on a final occasion the spirit said that she would not appear again.

Livermore was incredibly grateful to Kate and in 1871 paid for her to go to England. He felt that he did not wish her to go and receive payments for her work, but that she should regard herself as a spiritualist missionary, hence his willingness to subsidise her. In England she married H.D. Jencken, a prominent barrister and eager spiritualist, with whom she had two children. Over the years she conducted several séances under experimental conditions, convincing some ardent sceptics in the process.

Margaret joined Kate in England for a while and they always maintained cordial relations. This was not the case with their elder sister Leah, with whom they fell out dramatically in the late 1880s over a dispute about spiritualism. Seemingly both Kate and Margaret seemed to undergo a detestation of spiritualism, despite their prominence in the movement. At a public demonstration before the press in 1888 Margaret showed that she could at will produce the rapping noise by cracking the joints in her big toe.

One would have expected this to have had a devastating effect upon spiritualism, but it did not. It did destroy the two sisters' credibility and they were jettisoned by the movement, which still had strong affiliations with the temperance movement. It was said that alcohol had destroyed their judgement and that they had both fallen so low that they would do anything to feed their habit.

Sadly, both younger sisters sank into and died in poverty, both being buried in pauper's graves. Yet the spirit of spiritualism lived on.

MRS MARIA HAYDEN

There were several spiritualists who had come to Britain almost as soon as the Fox sisters had spearheaded the movement. They held meetings or gave séances at which they delivered messages from the other side of the misty veil – as the barrier between the living world and the spirit realm was known by them. One of the first spiritualists to gain celebrity and attract attention was Mrs Maria B. Hayden, the wife of the Boston journalist W.R. Hayden, who edited a newspaper called *The Boston Atlas* and also a monthly newsletter called *The Star Spangled Banner*. Like the Fox family they were ardent abolitionists. Although she is often credited as being the first person to bring spiritualism to Britain, she was in fact the first one to bring the rapping method.

In 1851 she and her husband invited Daniel Dunglas Home, one of the most famous and important Victorian-era spiritualists, to conduct a séance at their Connecticut home. We shall meet Home again soon; suffice it to say that he was only 18 at the time, but he impressed them immensely. Hayden wrote a glowing report about the séance in his newspaper, which certainly enhanced Home's reputation. Whether Mrs Hayden was aware of her ability then or not is unclear. What is known is that she was practising as a medium, specialising in rapping phenomena shortly afterwards.

In 1852 she and her husband came to England in the company of a Mr Stone, a lecturer and adept in 'electro-biology', one of the pseudo-scientific names for hypnosis at the time.

It is uncertain how old Mrs Hayden was when she arrived in England, but she is described as being young and vivacious, well educated and well mannered. There is some suggestion that she had the air of an adventuress about her. At any rate, she charmed people as she went about.

The newspapers had done a good job of advertising for her before she even arrived, so her reputation truly did go before her. Then once she had settled in she was eagerly sought out and put to the test. The first such occasion was at a séance in a house in Cavendish Square, which was attended by a small select group of the literati, including the publisher Robert Chambers and the novelist Mrs Catherine Crowe, the author of *The Night Side of Nature, or Ghosts and Ghost-seers*. This book was something of a nineteenth-century bestseller which examined the evidence about ghosts, apparitions, poltergeists, telepathy and psychic phenomena. The point is that these were people worth impressing and it seems that if Mrs Hayden did not impress them all she impressed some of them enough to stir up a whole series of invitations. Robert Chambers would not commit himself at the time, yet a couple of years later he was ready to support her.

Mrs Hayden's method involved the production of raps in answer to questions. Many people thought her method and her answers were wonderful, yet others said that she was only able to give coherent answers if she had sight of the alphabet. Robert Chambers asserted that he had seen her give unaccountably accurate answers even with the alphabet behind her back.

For several months she gave séances which were well attended and which only gathered favourable reviews. Then the sceptical ones started to roll off the press, notably with scathing pieces in *Blackwood's Magazine*, *Household Words* and *The National Miscellany*.

Despite this negativity she maintained a positive reputation and was instrumental in boosting converts to spiritualism. In this she was helped by her husband who put his journalistic expertise to good use and produced a magazine, *The Spirit World*, in 1853. It was the first spiritualist magazine in Britain and presumably he intended to run it for a long time. As it was, later in 1853 they decided to return to America.

There, Mrs Hayden studied medicine, graduated as a doctor and set up a highly successful practice. It seems that she had given up communicating with the spirit world.

MRS CORA SCOTT

A quite different pioneer of spiritualism was Cora L.V. Scott (1840–1923). She worked as an author of spiritualist literature and a trance medium, conveying messages from the spirit world whenever she was in a state of trance. She spent most of her life in America, but made three long trips to Britain after 1875. She was highly influential because of the type of messages that she gave.

Cora Scott was born in Cuba, NewYork in 1841. Her family were Presbyterians, but joined the Universalist Church in 1851. Essentially, they believed that everyone carried some original sin, but that everyone could achieve salvation. The principles of non-violence, abolition and temperance were highly regarded. Once again, this was fertile ground for a potential spiritualist.

Cora's full birth name was Cora Lodensia Veronika Scott, but she disliked her middle names and always called herself Cora L.V. Stunningly beautiful, she was to be married several times, on each occasion using the latest married surname. Thus she was at different times known as Cora L.V. Scott Hatch, or Daniels, or Tappan, or Richmond. She visited England twice as Mrs Cora Tappan and once during her honeymoon as Mrs Cora Richmond.

Her 'gift' was discovered at the age of 11 when she first fell into a trance and channelled spirits. Her parents began taking her on tours in the locality, where she would channel messages and give healing. By the age of 14 she was quite famous and her healing was done by psychic surgery, whereby she would channel the spirit of a German surgeon and psychically remove diseased parts from the patient's etheric body.

When she was about 15 the healing ability seemingly left her, or the German surgeon's spirit was no longer channelled through her. From then on she would give messages and also deliver lectures on various esoteric or philosophical subjects in a state of trance. Her ability under trance to speak so eloquently and seemingly totally unrehearsed convinced many who heard her that she had to be channelling, for it was considered implausible for one so young to be able to speak with such knowledge and authority. Later, she would transcribe lectures on spiritualism and became an author of a substantial body of work.

Her first husband, Benjamin Franklin Hatch, was a professional mesmerist and something of a showman. When they met he was a mere 16-year-old and he was 46. He managed her spiritualist career for several years until the marriage fell apart and they divorced.

In 1865 she moved to Washington and was apparently sought out for advice by several people who were in communication with President Lincoln about the current state of the Civil War that was raging.

President Ulysses S. Grant is said to have given her a Resolution of Gratitude for her support during his first administration.

In 1883 she visited Washington again and before a gathering gave a trance message, *A Message to the Nation*, purportedly channelled from the spirit of President James A. Garfield, who had been assassinated in 1881.

D.D. HOME

One of the most famous and influential spiritualists to cross the Atlantic to Britain was Daniel Dunglas Home (1833–86). He is often described as being an American spiritualist, yet he was in fact Scottish, having been born in Currie in Edinburgh. Seemingly gifted from a very early age, he was capable of producing all manner of psychic phenomena, from table tapping to clairvoyance, channelling and, most famously, levitation. His importance lies in the fact that although he gave several hundred séances to many people under strict conditions, he was never discovered to have used fraudulent methods.

Daniel was born of a family that contained several people who were reputed to have the gift of second sight, including his mother, Elizabeth. His father, David Home, was allegedly the illegitimate son of the 10th Earl of Home. He himself was the third of eight children and, as was not uncommon in those days, he was passed to his mother's childless sister Mary to be brought up. She and her husband immigrated to America in about 1840. Subsequently, his mother also immigrated and she was briefly reunited with Daniel. It was not to be for long, however, since she had a vision of her own death, which sadly proved to be accurate soon after.

Throughout his early years psychic phenomena happened around Daniel. Rather like the Fox sisters, there were frequent rappings and noises and movement of furniture. He also had visions, the second sight of the Homes, and on one occasion saw a vision of a close friend. It was found out that some days prior to Daniel's vision the friend had suddenly died.

We have already heard of how he gave his first séance at the home of the Hayden's. The publicity that he was then given by Mr Hayden catapulted him into the limelight and he toured near and far, giving readings and healing. Notably, he never claimed fees, but money in the form of gifts followed him everywhere.

Curiously, Daniel was by nature a shy man and professed a dislike of the limelight which his gift had thrust upon him. He travelled about the country, giving séances in New York, Boston and Newburgh. There he began to study medicine with the intention of building a medical practice. Unfortunately, he developed tuberculosis and was compelled to halt his studies. For the sake of his health he was advised to travel to Europe to convalesce. London and fame unimaginable beckoned him, although he did not know it at the time.

Before he arrived in England in 1855 he had used his full name, but from then on he became known as D.D. Home. Rather like Mrs Hayden, whom he may well have inspired, his fame preceded him and his arrival in London was eagerly awaited by those intrigued by spiritualism. He was fortunate in gaining patronage of a form straight away. This came in the form of free lodging at Cox's Hotel in Jermyn Street, the hotel owned by an enthusiastic spiritualist and hotel owner, William Cox. He was fortunate to receive similar offers of free accommodation, usually in some luxury, for the rest of his life.

D.D. Home, as we should now refer to him, was quite unique among spiritualist mediums, for he never gave public performances nor did he charge fees, ignoring the substantial gifts that came his way. His demonstrations of mediumship came about in private chambers, soirees and at parties. He never promised that phenomena would occur, since he averred that although he had powers, they were beyond his control. He could not deliberately exercise them.

So what were some of these phenomena? Well, by all accounts any manner of events could occur. They were only likely to do so, however, in subdued lighting, although he did not apparently ask for lights to be completely extinguished as did so many mediums of the day. Luminescent phenomena were common, as were rappings, table turning and channelling. Ectoplasmic appearances, one of the most desired psychic phenomena to occur, could happen. Ghostly hands could appear and touch people, objects could rise, drums could be played, instruments blown to make noises. There was also the possibility of ghostly writing appearing and of levitation of the medium himself.

He had his ardent believers, including Elizabeth Barrett Browning, John Ruskin, Anthony Trollope, Lord Lytton and the social reformer Robert Owen. Yet he also had vehement critics, such as the poet Robert Browning, Elizabeth's husband. The scientists Michael Faraday and Thomas Huxley were also extremely scathing, although they had no evidence that the things he produced were in any way fraudulent. Yet another eminent scientist, Sir William Crookes, the inventor of the Crookes tube and discoverer of several important phenomena in the fields of chemistry and spectroscopy, was a firm supporter, simply because he could find no way that Home could have falsified the things that happened.

Home's levitations became famous. During séances he would seemingly start to rise into the air, his voice moving ever upwards towards the ceiling, while witnesses could actually touch his feet to prove to themselves that he was floating upwards. This was not something that happened once or twice but, according to Crookes, over fifty times. Indeed, he said that he had been witnessed to levitate to a height of 6 or 7ft in 'good light'. By this it was meant gaslight. That may sound dubious, yet it is not as dubious as doing so in the dark when it would be possible to suspend shoes on poles and allow them to be felt.

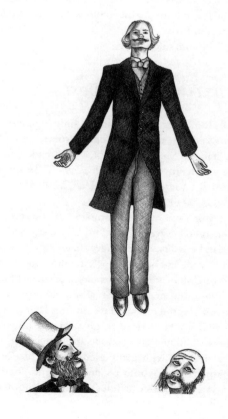

D.D. Home
apparently levitating.

His most famous levitation took place in 1868 at a house in Westminster in the presence of three stalwart young men. These were Viscount Adare, Lord Lindsay and a Captain Wynne. All three were regarded as good witnesses and all went on to hold positions of responsibility. Lindsay became President of the Royal Astronomical Society and Wynne became a magistrate.

The séance took place in a room on the third floor of a building. Home left the three men in one room and went into a neighbouring room. They heard a window being thrown open then a few moments later D.D. Home floated in through the open window of their room. A subsequent examination of the rooms and the walls convinced all three men that there was no way that he could have climbed out of or jumped the distance between the windows. Their only conclusion was that he must have been levitated or carried by outside forces from one room to the other.

Lindsay reported that this was not done in the darkness, but that '... the moon was shining full into the room'.

D.D. Home married twice. His first marriage was to the 17-year-old Russian Alexandra de Kroll, with whom they had a son. Sadly, she died shortly afterwards of tuberculosis. His second wife, Julie de Gloumeline, was a wealthy Russian lady who outlived him. He died from the tuberculosis that had plagued him at the age of 55 in some comfort in Paris.

His secrets went with him to the grave.

REVEREND WILLIAM STAINTON MOSES

Undoubtedly D.D. Home was instrumental in influencing several people who subsequently discovered that they had mediumistic talents. One such was the Reverend William Stainton Moses (1839–92), who attended one of his séances in the early 1870s. He was to prove to be a leading light in the spiritualist movement in the latter part of the Victorian era. Indeed, he may have been almost as successful and famed as D.D. Home.

William Stainton Moses was born in Donington in the county of Lincolnshire, the son of a schoolmaster. He went to Oxford University and was ordained into the Church of England in 1863. He had never been robust in health and in 1870 he gave up his parish work and became a private tutor. Shortly afterwards he was appointed as senior English master at University College School.

In 1872 he became interested in spiritualism and attended several séances, including one given by Home himself. Five months later he started to become aware of his own abilities. He started to give séances himself, to friends and associates. Soon, he was building up a considerable reputation.

As seemed to be the case with many mediums, he first became aware that he could contact spirits who would produce rapping phenomena and table turning. He reported that toilet articles in his bedroom would rearrange themselves as spirits sought to gain his attention. Then there were apports[4] of odours, pincushions and other small objects. Then lights would appear at his séances much to the amazement of the sitters. Levitation was a phenomenon that came relatively early to him. Apparently he would actually seem to rise and float about in his chair during séances.

Yet the most impressive of the phenomena that he produced were his automatic writings. In trance he would channel spirits who would direct him to write. Between 1872 and 1883 he filled twenty-four notebooks with writings. These messages were said to be from specific spirits, whom he called Imperator and Rector. These he published in the spiritualistic literature as *Spirit Teachings* and *Spirit Identity*. The essence of them was theological, implying that spiritualism was the truest and best religion for mankind to follow.

In 1878 he wrote a book, *Psychography, A Treatise on one of the Objective Forms of Psychic or Spiritual Phenomena*. In it he coined the word 'psychography', meaning, essentially, spirit writing. This was, of course, quite a different form of spirit writing than the production of actual pieces of writing as if they had been done by the spirits using pencil or slate, which other mediums did.

William was never discovered committing any fraud, although it is suggested that his spirit lights could have been chemically induced with phosphorescent substances. His character and his profession worked very much to his benefit in this, and he had many staunch followers and friends.

He was also involved in psychical research and was a member of the Psychological Society and later of the Society for Psychical Research, albeit not for long. In addition, he was a founding member of the British National Association of Spiritualists in 1882. We shall meet him again in Chapter 10 Ghost Hunters and Psychic Investigation.

DR HENRY SLADE

Another famous American spiritualist was Henry Slade (1839–1905). He specialised in the appearance of messages in chalk on writing slates or pencil on paper from his spirit guide, whom he claimed was his deceased wife. He styled himself Dr Henry Slade, although there is no evidence that he was eligible in any way to use the title. He achieved great success and fame in both the United States and Europe in the Victorian era.

According to William E. Robinson (who was latterly known to the world as 'The Marvellous Chinese Conjuror, Chung Ling Soo') in his book *Spirit Slate Writing and Kindred Phenomena*, 'no phenomenon which psychic mediums produced in the nineteenth century converted more persons to belief in spirits than the supposed writing by spirits on school slates'.

---

4. An apport was the production of aromas or of objects as diverse as flowers, thimbles or paper – apparently from the spirit realm.

Henry Slade was credited as being the first medium to have discovered the ability of the spirits to produce such messages.

Slade charged high fees for his psychic consultations, during which he would show a blank school slate on both sides, then concentrate and contact his spirit guide who would try to send a message. To receive it he would momentarily lower the slate under the consulting table, for as everyone was aware the spirits needed shade or darkness. Upon bringing it back the message would be there for anyone to read.

In 1876 Slade stopped in London en route to St Petersburg, where he was due to demonstrate his powers before Madame Helena Blavatsky and Colonel Harry Steel Olcott, who would soon afterwards co-found the Theosophical Society. While he was in London he entertained clients who were eager to receive a slate reading. Unfortunately for him he aroused the suspicions of one client who, together with a colleague, arranged a 'sting' operation whereby they discovered that he was deceiving them. It resulted in a famous court case in which the well-known magician John Nevil Maskelyne was called to give evidence.

Things went badly for Slade and he was found guilty of trying to accept money under false pretences. He was sentenced to three months' hard labour, but evaded imprisonment because of a technicality. He and his assistant absconded to France before a further proceeding could get underway.

The case did a great deal of harm to the spiritualist movement. On the other hand, it strengthened the reputation of Maskelyne, as we shall see in Chapter 14 The Egyptian Hall, in Part Three of the book, when we will look at the case in more detail.

QUEEN VICTORIA AND SPIRITUALISM

One of the greatest boosts to the spiritualist movement may actually have come from the reigning monarch herself. At least, that is the story that for many years was recounted in spiritualistic circles. It does indeed sound plausible, yet historians are unsure whether there is any real documentary evidence for it. The story goes that up until 1963 there was a gold watch displayed in the College of Psychic Studies in London.[5] A plaque explained that the watch was engraved:

> Presented by Her Majesty to Miss Georgiana Eagle for her Meritorious and Extraordinary Clairvoyance Produced at Osborn House, Isle of Wight, July 17, 1846.

The suggestion is that Queen Victoria was interested in occult matters and had received clairvoyant messages from a young girl, Georgiana Eagle. However, the

---

5. This organisation was founded in 1884 as the London Spiritualist Alliance. It is still very active and involved in psychic research.

fact is that the watch was stolen and has never been recovered. Also, there is no evidence that Georgiana ever existed. Could the watch have been a fake? If so, why was such a fake perpetrated?

Yet there is more, since it is also widely reported in spiritualistic literature that after the tragic death of Price Albert in 1861 Queen Victoria consulted the medium Robert James Lees (1849–1931) and had six séances with him, during which he contacted the spirit of her husband. Apparently, the spirit of Prince Albert gave her advice, much as he had done throughout their marriage. It is said that she later appointed Robert Lees to be her royal psychic. It is interesting to note that if it is true, he would only have been 12 years old at the time he started contacting Prince Albert's spirit for her.

Whether there is truth in it or not, the fact is that rumours spread, and rumour of royal patronage can do nothing but good for a movement.

Robert Lees went on to establish a lucrative and successful mediumship career. He was an adept spirit writer and later authored several spiritualistic texts which he claimed to have been channelled from the spirit world. He simply called himself 'The Recorder'.

In 1888, at the time of the Jack the Ripper murders in Whitechapel in London, Lees offered his services to Scotland Yard. The official version is that they turned him away, thinking that he was insane. Fictionalised versions in books and film suggest that Lees actually was a gifted medium. Perhaps he was, but we shall never know.

9

PSYCHIC PHENOMENA AND SÉANCES

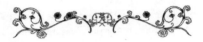

It is wonderful that five thousand years have now elapsed since the creation of the
world, and still it is undecided whether or not there has ever been an instance of the
spirit of any person appearing after death. All argument is against it; but all belief is
for it.

Dr Samuel Johnson

Victorians went to spiritualist meetings in order to receive messages from the
spirit world. In the early days, mediums held public meetings in halls and large
venues with the medium on stage, either receiving messages while in trance or
in a state of clear consciousness. It was actually at séances, often in the medium's
home or in private residences, when most of the spectacular psychic phenomena
occurred. The word séance actually came from old French for seat or sitting.

We tend to think of Victorian séances being conducted round a table. This
indeed was often the case, the sitters forming a ring and touching hands. Most
often the lights would be dimmed or even completely extinguished, for it was
said that the spirits did not like the light. The medium would either remain in
consciousness or, more usually, drift off into a trance of some sort when they
would make contact with one spirit control in particular, or channel messages
from spirits who had specifically come there in the spirit world to give a message
to a sitter.

As the spiritualist movement developed it became apparent that mediums
tended to concentrate on their own method. Some, such as the Fox sisters and
Mrs Hayden, would use a method of table rapping; others would go into a trance
and produce messages, like Cora L.V. Scott. Others would induce the spirits to
move objects, while some would produce writing, or cause spirits to manifest
themselves as lights or as some form of ectoplasm.

Some mediums claimed affiliation with a particular type of religion, while others gradually formed themselves into a formal religion, the mediums becoming ordained preachers or ministers of the religion. Cora L.V. Scott, for example, founded her Church of the Soul in Chicago, where she gave weekly services and trance readings.

David Richmond of Darlington in 1853 opened the Spiritualist Church in England, having discovered spiritualism on a trip to the United States. Others followed and there were several spiritualist churches dotted around the country by 1870. Most did not have a central method of worship as did other religions, but would hold meetings that would be determined by whatever type of medium had been invited to attend. Thus D.D. Home on occasions shared meetings with Kate Fox in London.

People were attracted to spiritualism in its broadest sense for different reasons. The majority were people who had been bereaved and who sought some means of salving the pain of their grief and hoped to get some sort of message from their loved ones, be that a child, a parent or a partner. These were days of early and often painful deaths when infant mortality was high and medicine had little to offer against many of the infectious diseases, and was of virtually no help in treating malignant conditions.

A large number of people were simply questioning whether or not they could receive evidence that there was life after death. If so, it would be immensely comforting and in a way would make sense for the hardships and drudgery of the lives they had to endure.

Still others were simply curious and looked upon spiritualism as a sort of entertainment. This latter group tended to belong to the more leisured upper and upper-middle classes who had what the lower classes did not have – leisure. And so dabbling in spiritualism at afternoon tea parties became a social phenomenon. Tea, cakes and some conversation may be followed by a light-hearted séance or a little experiment with table rapping, table turning or trying to communicate with the spirits via a planchette or spirit writing.

There were also those who wished to seriously examine the phenomena that the various mediums claimed to produce. Their purpose was entirely scientific and we shall consider them further in Chapter 11 Ghost Hunters and Psychic Investigation.

Finally, there was a group of people who were completely sceptical of the majority of, if not all, mediums, whom they suspected were simply out to dupe the bereaved and the grief-stricken. In their eyes these people were nothing but charlatans who had to be exposed. This was not a large group, but it was one with some expertise in deception, for they were themselves professional magicians. We shall introduce them in this chapter, but consider some of their concerns later in Part Three.

PSYCHIC PHENOMENA

As we saw in the last chapter, Kate Fox married the barrister H.R. Jencken in 1871. He was somewhat concerned about the hotchpotch of practices and phenomena that different mediums were producing, and he saw that there was a need for clarification and some categorisation. He therefore produced a list of the sort of phenomena that could be encountered at séances. Thus:

> The movement and raising of ponderable bodies, including levitation of the medium
> The production of raps and knocks
> The uttering of words, sentences, sounding of music, singing, imitation of birds
> Playing on musical instruments, the drawing of flowers, figures, and writing by
>   direct spiritual unseen agency
> The fire test
> Elongation of the medium's body
> Holding fluids in space without bottles or containers, the perfuming of water, the
>   extraction of scent from flowers, or alcohol from spirits of wine

All of these had been reported on over the relatively short period of time that spiritualism had been in existence. We heard a little about it in the last chapter, but it is interesting to look at some of the reported sightings of these phenomena since the written word was the Victorians' main source of information, apart from direct viewing of a medium at work. This is quite important, actually, since one should never underestimate the power and influence of the written word. There is, after all, much truth in the old axiom that the pen is mightier than the sword. Of course, with such a contentious subject as spiritualism there would be much thrust and counter-thrust in the newspapers and periodicals.

It is also worth noting that over time there had been a general change in the type of activity that mediums elicited. At first it tended to be simple table rapping or table turning. Then materialisations started to be used, at first in the form of light phenomena, then later in the production of images and even of physical things. As we shall see, these increasingly physical manifestations were less and less plausible, yet more and more dramatic, as competition among mediums started to develop.

Natural scepticism among sitters resulted in their need to ensure that the mediums were actually producing phenomena and not simply tricking them. Accordingly, whereas mediums like Mrs Hayden had been able to conduct their séances unfettered later mediums had to conduct their séances while they were held, tied or even chained up. Many had to endure body searches for hidden apparatus or paraphernalia with which they could produce ghostly phenomena.

We will have a look at some of the phenomena first, and then focus on some interesting mediums who were right at the interface between mediumship and magicianry: the Davenport brothers.

RAPPING

This was really the first phenomenon to be used, as was demonstrated by the Fox sisters. The noises could vary immensely from thuds to raps, to creaks. The fact that they had no apparent physical cause, but came in answer to questions, was the important thing. That made people believe that there were answers coming from the other side.

TABLE LIFTING AND TABLE TURNING

These are two interesting physical phenomena that became extremely common at séances. Sitters would sit round a table with their hands on the table, each person touching the fingers of the person next to them. As the séance progressed the spirits would be contacted and the table would either lift or begin to turn. Sometimes it would be a mere tilting, sometimes violently and sometimes just with a steady pressure so that the table would rise into the air, pushing upwards into the sitters' hands.

There were different ways of doing a table–lifting séance. The sitters could ask questions and receive 'yes' or 'no' answers by the table lifting a certain number of times. Letters of the alphabet could be laid or drawn around the table, usually a round table, and the table would be turned as the letters were spelled out.

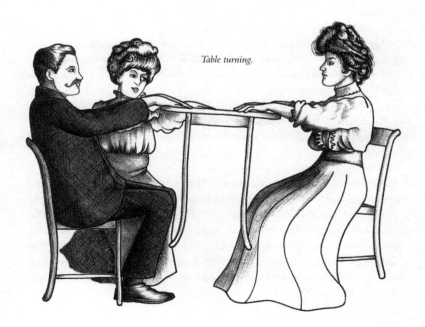

Table turning.

LEVITATION

The raising of objects on the table in a dimly lit séance room would have been impressive for most people. Sitters would see tambourines rise and shake, handkerchiefs, books and drums rise into the air and dance about. So too would things jump or seem to be thrown around. Nothing, of course, was as impressive as being present when the medium was actually levitated.

A medium called Henry Gordon was apparently the first medium to levitate himself in 1853. His levitations were not, however, as impressive as those of D.D. Home.

MUSIC PHENOMENA

The medium D.D. Home recorded in his autobiography *Incidents of My Life* that he had been able to produce music for much of his life:

> At night when I was asleep my room would be filled with sounds of harmony, and these gradually grew louder until people in other parts of the house could hear them distinctly; if by any chance I awoke the music would instantly cease.

According to E.W. Capron's book *Modern Spiritualism*, published in 1855, a woman called Mrs Tamlin was the first medium to channel music from a musical instrument:

> In her presence it was played with all the exactness of an experienced musician, although she is not acquainted with music, or herself able to play any instrument. The tones varied from loud and vigorous to the most refined touches of the strings that could be imagined.

The naturalist Alfred Russel Wallace recorded that at the first séance by D.D. Home he attended he witnessed an accordion being played, seemingly by an outside agency:

> As I was the only one of the company who had not witnessed any of the remarkable phenomena that occurred in his presence, I was invited to go under the table while an accordion was playing, held in Home's hand, his other hand being on the table. The room was well lighted and I distinctly saw Home's hand holding the instrument which moved up and down and played a tune without any visible cause. He then said, "Now I will take away my hand," which he did, but the instrument went on playing and I saw a detached hand holding it while Home's two hands were seen above the table by all present.

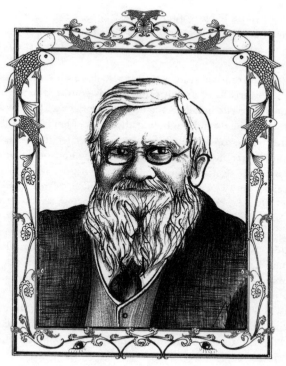

Alfred Russel Wallace.

MATERIALISATION

This was a phenomenon that occurred more frequently as spiritualism developed. It was often dramatic, in that images of people, or of ghostly body parts, would appear during a séance. So dramatic was it that people would visit mediums just to see such a thing or, better still, be able to touch it. Understandably, such manifestations seemingly from the spirit world could often cause intense anxiety and fear in people of a nervous disposition.

Ghostly translucent hands would appear, reach out and touch people to make their hair stand on end. Or they would appear from under the table to touch a sitter and make them scream. Then they would disappear without a trace. These were always impressive and it was not until years later when magicians like Robert-Houdin, Harry Kellar and, later still, Harry Houdini demonstrated how to create such spirit hands from wax.

Florence Cook (1856–1904) was to become the most famous of the materialisation mediums. She had been 'trained' by Frank Herne, another physical medium. He had a spirit control who guided him in his work and it seems that under his influence she discovered that she too had a spirit by the name of Katie

King. Now this Katie King is interesting because she did not appear to be a spirit exclusively attached to Florence Cook. She had seemingly attached herself temporarily to other mediums, but it was to Florence that she seemed most attracted or attached.

Florence conducted her séances in the usual way but also made use of a common mediumistic tool, a spirit cabinet. This consisted of a cupboard into which the medium went, usually being bound in some way. Florence had a large cupboard in which she sat and was bound, the knots of her bindings being sealed. Through a hole at the top of the cabinet she would materialise veiled spirit faces. Later, she would materialise the spirit of Katie King, who would leave the cabinet and actually enter the séance room.

At one séance, on 9 December 1873, Katie King appeared in white flowing garments and left the cabinet. Unbeknown to Florence there was a rival medium, William Volckman, present at the séance, and he suddenly jumped up and attempted to seize the spirit. Other sitters wrestled him, causing him some injury, which included tearing out some of his beard. He claimed that Florence was a fake, yet when the lights went up and the spirit cabinet was opened they found Florence somewhat agitatedly sitting there, her sealed bindings intact. Of the 'spirit clothes' there was no sign.

Florence Cook's reputation took a hammering that night, although she still maintained a large following. Interestingly, William Volckman later married another of Florence Cook's rivals, the medium Mrs Guppy, of whom we shall learn more shortly.

APPORTS

These also became more common as mediums moved away from the table rapping of the early mediums. An 'apport' was the name given to an object that materialised during a séance. It could take the form of plants, animals, birds or common or garden objects. Often someone other than the medium would make a suggestion in the séance and the appropriate apport would appear.

Mrs Agnes Nichol Guppy (1833–1917) was one of the most famous physical mediums of the Victorian era. By this it is meant that she specialised in physical phenomena. She had been discovered by Alfred Russel Wallace at the home of his sister, Mrs Sims, in 1866. She was a large woman who made a living as a professional hypnotist and medium. She had a reputation for being able to shift furniture and table-turn. Wallace followed her development closely and witnessed several levitations of her during séances. He also apparently saw her produce apports in the form of nettles, flowers and fruits.

Many mediums followed suit and physical apports became quite commonplace. But Mrs Guppy became famous for another thing that she could do – transportation.

TRANSPORTATION

This phenomenon was a form of apportation, in that objects were transported from one place into the séance. This could be from a great distance away. Nothing, however, could be more dramatic that the transportation of a medium, and that is just what Mrs Guppy is alleged to have done.

On the 3 June 1871 a séance was held by ten people at 61 Lamb's Conduit Street, 3 miles from the Highbury home of Mrs Guppy, where she was apparently relaxing in the evening by doing some writing before retiring for the night. The people present at the séance included two mediums, Charles Williams and Frank Herne, and eight sitters. Someone made a humorous request that it would be good to have Mrs Guppy present. To their immense surprise, three minutes later something heavy thumped into the séance table. A match was struck and everyone gasped to find Mrs Guppy had been transported in a state of trance and half-dress right into their midst.

ELONGATION

The same Frank Herne was the first medium to demonstrate elongation of a limb. He claimed to have a spirit control who was the long-dead pirate Sir Henry Morgan. At the home of a Dr Dixon in 1871 he apparently demonstrated that his body could be stretched to a great degree through the aid of his spirit control.

SPIRIT WRITING

This became very popular and took several forms. The first type was a physical phenomenon in which a message would physically appear written in chalk on slates, or in pencil on paper, or sometimes in luminescent ink. The second would be automatic writing, in which a medium would go into a trance and channel a spirit who would direct the medium's hand to produce a message.

Spirit writing with a planchette.

Henry Slade (1835–1905) was a famous medium who specialised in producing spirit messages on slate. The magician John Nevil Maskelyne was instrumental in exposing him and having him sentenced to three months' imprisonment.

THE PLANCHETTE

This was a small board usually shaped like a heart so one end had a pointer. It was mounted on two small castors and had a hole in it with a downturned pencil, which acted as a third castor. The idea was that the medium, or the sitters at the séance, would place fingers on it and it would slide around, the pencil writing a message.

It was apparently first used by a French medium called Monsieur Planchette in the early nineteenth century. It is not certain whether there actually was such a person, since the word in French means 'small plank'. Nevertheless, it is possible, as it could have been a stage name, such as the ones magicians would use.

The planchette was also often used to simply indicate letters of the alphabet, numbers or the answers 'yes' and 'no', which were laid out on a board. As such this was developed into the Ouija board.

THE SPIRIT IN THE GLASS

A popular method of contacting the spirits was easily done at impromptu séances across the country. An upturned glass would be used to indicate letters and numbers that were placed around a table. The sitters would each place a finger on the glass and could each ask questions, which, if they successfully contacted a spirit, would be spelled out.

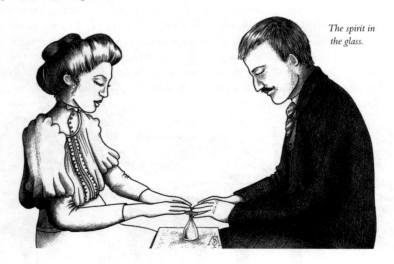

The spirit in the glass.

SPIRIT CONTROLS

Many mediums claimed to have one spirit in particular who acted as a regular guide for them in the spirit world. Florence Cook, for example, said that she had been aware of a spirit girl who had once lived in the living world as Annie Morgan, but who was known in the spirit world as Katie King. She was her regular control spirit or guide and would appear at materialisations.

It was also said that spirit controls could manifest themselves to other mediums. Indeed, Katie King's father, William King, was another spirit who would apparently frequently pop up at séances held by other mediums. They became famous, and in a way added to the credibility of other mediums who were able to attract them at their séances.

SPIRIT PHOTOGRAPHY

This was a development that occurred during the Victorian era as the new science of photography developed. To be able to actually photograph a spirit during a séance was thought to be a way of scientifically proving that spirits existed, and, therefore, that a medium had the power to bring back the dead in a form that could be seen.

The first spirit photograph was produced by a photographer called Mumler, in Boston, United States, in 1862. He took a photograph of a Dr Gardner, who when he saw the plate identified a spirit likeness of his cousin who had died twelve years previously. Dr Gardner published the photograph, which was haled as a breakthrough for spiritualism.

A year later, Dr Gardner discovered that at least two spirit photographs taken by Mumler showed images of live people that he had taken separately.

Six years after that Mumler moved to New York and again started to produce spirit photographs. The authorities attempted to prosecute him, but were unsuccessful since they had no hard evidence.

Mr and Mrs Guppy were among the first mediums to try to introduce spirit photography to Britain. They tried to do it themselves, but lacked experience in photography. They then began working with a photographer called Hudson, who was able to capture Mrs Guppy and one of her materialisations on a plate. It was the beginning of a great success for Mr Hudson, who did a booming trade.

Inevitably, there were sceptics and Hudson was investigated. Mr Trail Taylor, the editor of the *British Journal of Photography*, witnessed him taking a spirit photograph. He was totally convinced of its authenticity.

THE DAVENPORT BROTHERS

In 1864 two young American brothers arrived in London and immediately set about causing a stir. They proved to be something of an enigma in the history of spiritualism, for although the phenomena that they produced were purported to be the result of spirit action, they themselves never claimed to have special powers. They did not have to; they had people about them who did.

Ira (1839–1911) and William (1841–77) Davenport had a similar history to that of the Fox sisters, in that from an early age mysterious rappings and noises had been reported around them when they were children. Almost inevitably people took an avid interest in them, for news of spiritualism was spreading like wildfire. They quickly developed a routine that convinced people that they were especially gifted mediums.

At first they were managed by their father, who had retired from the New York police force in order to look after their interests. Then they were joined by a Nonconformist minister, Dr J.B. Ferguson, who proclaimed that they had been given a divine gift, the purpose of which was to show people the power of God and to enlighten them about the world of spirit. For ten years they toured America, the centre feature of their act being a huge spirit cabinet.

Their performance was generally done in the round, in that people would sit in a large ring around them, holding hands to ensure that no one aided them. The brothers entered the cabinet and were securely tied up and the doors closed. Then the phenomena began. A variety of musical instruments were played, tambourines were shaken, bells rang and things were thrown out of the cabinet. Then, when the cabinet was opened, they were revealed to be securely tied.

It is perhaps a little surprising that this caused so much of a sensation, since it would seem obvious that they were adept at escapology, yet such was the interest in the occult and in spiritualism that people were willing to believe the things that Dr Ferguson told them. They were even more convinced when a spectator was tied inside the cabinet with the brothers, but still the phenomena occurred.

After the spirit cabinet antics had been performed they went on to perform outside the cabinet. They would be tied to chairs, away from a table on which a variety of things were placed. The lights would go down and the mysterious playing, throwing and spirit writing would occur. When the lights went back on the brothers were found exactly as before, tied to their chairs.

Their tour of the provinces did not go down as well as their London ventures. In Liverpool and Huddersfield spectators actually smashed the cabinet. And then the magicians moved in to expose them, but that is a tale that we will keep until Chapter 14 The Egyptian Hall.

10

MATERIALISATION

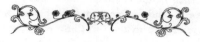

I think a Person who is thus terrified with the Imagination of Ghosts and Spectres much more reasonable, than one who contrary to the Reports of all Historians sacred and profane, ancient and modern, and to the Traditions of all Nations, thinks the Appearance of Spirits fabulous and groundless.

The Spectator, 1711
Joseph Addison

Nothing could convince people more than actual demonstrations of the presence of spirits. Materialisation of spirit hands, faces or even whole forms were performed at séances across the United States, Britain and Europe. These other-world manifestations varied immensely. Sometimes they were described as being wraith-like wisps of smoke, or gossamer-thin material like muslin. Faces were often static images surrounded by the transparent material, but at other times fully formed hands, feet, heads or even whole figures would appear. In the early days of spiritualism, before restrictions or tests were imposed on mediums, 'spirits' would move around the séance parlour.

Sitters were often invited to touch spectral hands, or were touched by them. Hair might be left by a spirit or a spirit might blow upon someone.

Sitters were discouraged from touching apparitions unless invited to do so, since it was not considered safe for the medium, who was usually in a state of trance, to have their spirit tampered with. The explanation, of course, was that they were acting as a conduit or channel between the world of the living and the dead; any interference could result in a medium collapsing or even suffering a near fatal injury. As far as the author is aware, however, no medium ever did expire during a materialisation séance.

SPIRIT CABINETS

It seems a curious thing to do, but mediums would sit in a cupboard or cabinet while the sitters would remain outside, holding hands. A few hymns may have been sung and then phenomena would start to occur. In a materialisation either faces would appear in a cut-out window of the cabinet, or a spirit form would come out of the cabinet and move around in the darkened parlour. Usually, they were described as being like living people swathed in white veils or white drapery.

Clearly, the sceptical view would be that the figure was simply the medium draped in muslin or other transparent drapery to disguise themselves. Accordingly, it became the practice to bind the medium so that this possibility was removed. In addition, often a sitter was invited to sit in the cabinet as well as to remove any other chance of shenanigans by the medium. As we saw in Chapter 8, the medium Florence Cook was exposed by one of her sitters, who happened to be the partner of a rival medium.

Mediums were often investigated by people unwilling to accept the veracity of their phenomena and there were several cases of muslin, false hair, wigs and other 'spirit' trappings being found in their belongings.

Florence Cook was not the only medium to have her 'spirit' grabbed and held, only to prove to be none other than the medium. The conclusion, one would think, would be totally damning, yet many spiritualists accounted for it by explaining that when a spirit manifested itself, it did so by using some of the vital energy of the medium. Therefore, the medium and the spirit would be linked by psychic threads. Thus a spirit could emerge from the cabinet, walk around the room, touch or even communicate with the sitters, before returning to the cabinet and to the medium to be absorbed into the medium's vital energy again. Conversely, if the spirit was interfered with and held, the psychic threads could result in the medium's physical body being pulled from the cabinet to materialise where the spirit had been!

BARON CARL VON REICHENBACH AND ODIC FORCE

During the Victorian era there was only a very flimsy explanation of how materialisations could be produced. Some 'substance' was needed to explain these unworldly phenomena.

A notable scientist in the Victorian era was Baron Carl von Reichenbach (1788–1869). He was a chemist, physicist, geologist, metallurgist and philosopher. His studies ranged far and wide across the sciences and he made several important discoveries, including that of paraffin and the development of kreosote. This latter discovery was of immense economic importance because it meant that there was a way of preserving wood out of doors.

His researches in magnetism and electricity and his philosophical leanings led him to wonder whether there could be another intangible force at work in nature which could explain life itself. He therefore came up with the concept of Odyle or Odic Force, a vital force, which permeated all living things. This he believed could be seen as a sort of aura by people who were especially sensitive. He also felt that this explained the phenomenon of mesmerism, or hypnosis.

The spiritualists were quick to take up the concept of Odyle, for if it was the force of life, that which animated the body, then when it departed the body it would enter the world of the spirit. It was an explanation, therefore, of the wraith-like materialisations that the mediums could produce.

ECTOPLASM

Not all materialisations were done with the medium separated from the sitters in a spirit cabinet. Many were done with the medium actually sitting as part of the séance circle. More often than not these were conducted in darkness or subdued light and a strange substance would begin to materialise from the medium's body. There are many descriptions of this in the early spiritualism literature. It was sometimes said to be semi-luminous or phosphorescent, vaporous, fluid-like, or diaphanous. It could come from the medium's mouth, nose, ears or from their body. Some of the descriptions are not very convincing, since they say that it came like wisps of muslin, or that the medium, in trance, pulled it from under their clothes. Nevertheless, countless people saw these materialisations and were deeply convinced that they were witnessing the entry of dead spirits from the other side.

The word 'ectoplasm' was not actually used until after the Victorian era. It was coined by Charles Richet, a physiologist when he was president of the Society for

Ectoplasmic spirits were frequent visitors at Victorian séances.

Psychical research. He was to be awarded the 1913 Nobel Prize for Medicine and Physiology. He derived the word from the Greek *ektos*, meaning 'outside', and *plasma*, meaning 'something moulded'. It perfectly describes what people seemed to be witnessing and was in-keeping with scientific thinking. It certainly gave mediums an opportunity to use quasi-scientific language in describing their materialisations.

THE MATERIALISATION SPECIALISTS

There are several mediums whose names stand out as specialists in materialisation.

Madame d'Esperance (1855–1916)

This lady, whose real name was Elizabeth Hope, became one of the most famous mediums of the Victorian era, both for her materialisations and her apports of flowers.

Her story is fairly typical of that of many mediums. She was aware of voices or presences in her less than happy childhood. (This makes one wonder whether the start of her mediumship was through that common childhood experience of having an imaginary friend who helps make the unbearable reality more pleasant.) In any case, the climate was ripe by the 1870s for her to develop her skills. She changed her name to Madame d'Esperance and started to give séances. Also in common with other mediums histories, it seemed that her skills developed from rappings and table turning to physical materialisations. The more adept she became the more fame she attracted, with the result that she was able to go on tour, taking her séances all over Europe.

Madame d'Esperance had several spirit controls. She had a male control called Walter Stacey, who was later joined by Yolande, an Arabian beauty, and Nepenthes an Egyptian princess. These entities would materialise at séances and were greeted with great enthusiasm by her sitters.

She would later write of her experiences in her book *Shadow Land*, published in 1897. In it she recounts the description of a materialisation at one of her séances given by one of her sitters:

> First a filmy, cloudy patch of something white is observed on the floor in front of the cabinet. It then gradually expands, visibly extending itself as if it were an animated patch of muslin, lying fold upon fold, on the floor, until extending about two and a half by three feet, and having a depth of a few inches – perhaps six or more. Presently it begins to rise slowly in or near the centre, as if a human head were underneath it, while the cloudy film on the floor begins to look more like muslin falling into folds about the portion so mysteriously rising. By the time it has attained two or more feet it looks as if a child were under it, and moving its arms about in all directions, as if manipulating something underneath. It continues

rising, sometimes sinking somewhat to rise again higher than before, until it attains a height of about five feet, when its form can be seen as if arranging the folds of drapery about its figure. Presently the arms rise considerably above the head and open outwards through a mass of cloud-like spirit drapery, and Yolande stands before us unveiled, graceful and beautiful, nearly five feet in height, having a turban-like head-dress, from beneath which her long black hair hangs over her shoulders and down her back. The superfluous white, veil-like drapery is wrapped round her for convenience, or thrown down on the carpet, out of the way till required again. All this occupies from ten to fifteen minutes to accomplish.

In her book she discussed the outrageous things that she had to endure when she was demonstrating in front of psychic researchers. In the Victorian era, complete with its self-conscious prudishness, having to be searched for props or fraud was an occupational hazard that mediums of both sexes had to endure.

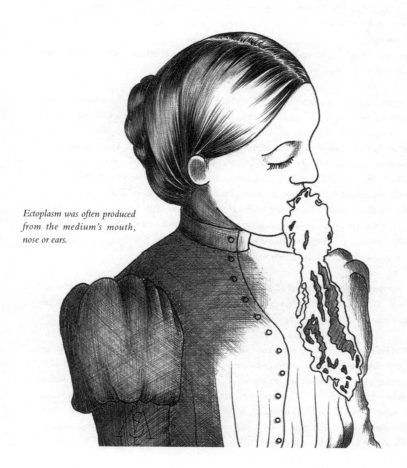

Ectoplasm was often produced from the medium's mouth, nose or ears.

William Eglinton (1858–1933)

Equal in fame to Madame d'Esperance was William Eglinton, who actually convinced Prime Minister William Gladstone of the reality of psychic phenomena and of the spirit world.

William Eglinton did not hear voices in his childhood. Indeed, he rather made fun of his father's interest in spiritualism, to the extent of pinning a derogatory and sarcastic notice on the door of the room in which he and friends were holding a séance. His father was furious and told him in no uncertain manner to either join them and see for himself or make himself scarce. He chose to stay.

According to William he intended to show that it was all nonsense, yet inexplicably the séance table started to move, totally beyond his control. He joined more séances and found that he could put himself into a state of trance during which phenomena would occur. During one such trance he was greeted by a spirit called Joey Sandy, who would become the first of his spirit controls.

Gradually the phenomena progressed through the ranks of rappings and table turning to levitation of himself and spirit materialisations. He quickly turned professional.

In 1885 a Mr Edmund Rogers described a materialisation during one of Eglinton's séances:

> He began gently to draw from his side and play out at right angles a dingy, white-looking substance, which fell down at his left side. The mass of white material on the floor increased in breadth, commenced to pulsate and move up and down, also swaying from side to side, the motor power being underneath. The height of this substance increased to about three feet, and shortly afterwards the 'form' quickly and quietly grew to its full stature. By a quick movement of his hand Mr. Eglinton drew away the white material which covered the head of the 'form' and it fell back over the shoulders and became part of the clothing of the visitor. The connecting link (the white appearance issuing from the side of the medium) was severed or became invisible, and the 'form' advanced to Mr. Everitt, shook hands with him, and passed round the circle, treating nearly everyone in the same manner.

He did not confine himself to spirit manifestations indoors. While staying with a Dr and Mrs Nichols in Malvern he conducted several séances, apparently under conditions controlled by Dr Nichols. The doctor described one:

> Mr. Eglinton lay on a garden bench in plain sight. We saw the bodies of four visitors form themselves from a cloud of white vapour and then walk about, robed all in purest white, upon the lawn where no deception was possible. One of them walked quite around us, as we sat in our chairs on the grass, talking as familiarly as any friend ... [and] took my hat from my head, put it on his own, and walked off with it where the medium was lying; then he came and put it on my head again; then walked across the lawn and up a gravel walk to the foot of the balcony and talked with

Mrs. Nichols. After a brief conversation he returned to the medium and gradually faded from sight.

Joey Sandy was not his only control. He also claimed to have a one-armed spirit control called Abdullah. He would materialise and appear in a turban with exotic jewels, which he would permit to be examined.

All did not go well with Eglinton, however, and he was exposed by the Archdeacon Thomas Colley. At a séance he had cut a piece of beard and a piece from a robe of a materialised spirit. These pieces were found to exactly fit a false beard and a muslin robe later found in Eglinton's possessions. The medium was out of the country at the time. An investigation was called for by the British National Association of Spiritualists, but no conclusion was reached since no hard evidence was produced. Presumably it had been spirited away!

Eglinton was examined on several occasions by members of the Society for Psychical Research, including Alfred Russel Wallace. Wallace was totally convinced of the genuineness of Abdullah's materialisation and did not think that there was any way in which the medium could have faked it.

Perhaps the intensity of the scrutiny that the Society for Psychical Research brought to bear on their investigations proved too much for him, for he then turned his attention to spirit slate reading. At a séance in 1884, attended by William Gladstone, he used slates owned by the séance hostess to produce messages in a variety of languages, including Greek and Spanish. The statesman was hugely impressed and as a result actually joined the Society for Psychical Research himself.

There was another significant event in Eglinton's mediumship career that we shall consider in Chapter 12 Theosophy.

Eusapia Palladino (1854–1918)

This Italian medium from Naples became famous for a variety of phenomena that she would produce at séances all over Europe and Russia. She was to be one of the most extensively investigated mediums. Her séances were investigated in 1892 in Milan by Professor Charles Richet and Cesare Lombroso, a prominent scientist. She completely convinced Lombroso of her abilities to the extent that he converted to spiritualism.

In Paris in 1903 Pierre and Marie Curie, both Nobel Prize winners, examined her and got her to perform séances under their control. Although she did not convince them, they could not detect any falsehood.

That is not to say that no one failed to detect any fraud. Indeed, she was caught on several occasions. Among the things that were discovered at séances in England, France and the United States were instances of her removing her feet from her shoes to producing table rapping; using hairs to make objects move; materialising spirit shapes by wrapping a handkerchief around her hand; producing rappings by clicking finger joints; and making a table levitate by using her foot and hand.

Despite all of these exposures she retained an amazingly loyal following. Even eminent researchers, such as Richet and Sir Oliver Lodge, refused to be persuaded that she was a perpetrator of fraudulent mediumship. And perhaps her most famous supporter, the creator of Sherlock Holmes, Sir Arthur Conan Doyle, utterly refused to believe that she was not entirely genuine.

ENCOURAGING BELIEF

Practicing as a professional medium gradually became more difficult as psychic investigators started using conjurors or seeking their opinions about how various phenomena could be produced. Because of that, materialisation mediumship became less common as the century entered its latter stages. Thus there seems to have been a shift in emphasis towards the production of other phenomena, such as spirit writing, direct channelling of spirits and the use of the medium's vocal cords to produce spirit voices.

Yet ardent spiritualists were always ready to have a materialisation. Mediums probably became very adept at detecting people who would be less vigilant in their scrutiny of what was going on. Credulous people, in other words, who fostered a believing attitude – an open-mindedness. This is encapsulated in the words of Edward Augustus Brackett in his 1885 book *Materialised Apparitions*:

> The key that unlocks the glories of another life is pure affection, simple and confiding as that which prompts the child to throw its arms around its mother's neck. To those who pride themselves upon their intellectual attainments, this may seem to be a surrender of the exercise of what they call the higher faculties. So far from this being the case, I can truly say that until I adopted this course, sincerely and without reservation, I learned nothing about these things. Instead of clouding my reason and judgment, it opened my mind to a clearer and more intelligent perception of what was passing before me. That spirit of gentleness, of loving kindness, which more than anything else crowns with eternal beauty the teachings of the Christ, should find its full expression in our association with these beings.

In essence, it was just what the spiritualist mediums asked of their sitters: to believe.

11

GHOST HUNTERS AND PSYCHIC INVESTIGATION

Now it is the time of night
That the graves, all gaping wide,
Every one lets forth his sprite
In the church-way paths to glide.

A Midsummer Night's Dream
William Shakespeare

Although the subtitle of this book is *The Victorian Age of Credulity*, that is not to say that all Victorians were credulous or gullible. Of course they were not, it is just that for any trend, movement or practice to become widespread there has to be a groundswell of opinion. A lot of people have to believe in it or be persuaded that there is something in it. That number has to grow, because once it recedes, it indicates that the trend is no longer credible for most people.

If people had been happy to just believe in the spirit world then the spiritualist movement would have continued to grow to become a major religion. It does still exist, of course, but not in the dubious form that it did in Victorian days. Nowadays mediums do not claim to produce ectoplasm, conjure up spirits to rattle tambourines, write spirit messages or cause objects to levitate. They do claim to channel spirits and communicate with the world of spirit, and it has to be said that they may very well be able to do so. Certainly many people attend spiritualist churches and are said to receive messages from the other side. There is no issue with this, since everyone is entitled to their belief and for those people who attend bona fide spiritualist churches and groups they may well be satisfied that their belief in the spirit world is being proven every time that a message is received.

Fraudulent mediumship, however, is another matter. It is that which scientists, magicians and psychic investigators sought to expose, because fraudulent mediums were simply being dishonest. They were playing with emotions and they were coining in a great deal of money and gaining fame in the process.

CATHERINE CROWE (1790–1872)

In the nineteenth century the name Catherine Crowe was well known. She was an acclaimed novelist and playwright, although her works have long since been forgotten. A non-fiction book that she wrote, *The Night Side of Nature, or Ghosts and Ghost-seers*, went on to be a Victorian bestseller and preceded the rise in spiritualism. It was published in 1848 and was an exhaustive investigation into ghosts, apparitions, poltergeists, telepathy and psychic phenomena.

Catherine was born in 1790 in Borough Green, Kent. She married Major John Crowe, an army officer seven years her senior, and they had one son. It was not a happy marriage, however, and they separated. She moved to Edinburgh and settled into the company of fellow writers. She also became friends with the philosopher and phrenologist George Combe, whom we met in Chapter 5 on phrenology. Understandably, she became fascinated by phrenology and the study of other outré subjects.

In 1841 she wrote a highly successful novel entitled *The Adventures of Susan Hopley*. It was the first of a series of social novels dealing with the subjugated position of women in society. Susan Hopley, her protagonist, is a servant and it is a story involving murder and duplicity. Early in the book she has a clairvoyant dream, in which she sees the murder of her master and her brother. This is interesting because it is indicative of Catherine's own interest in the occult.

The Night Side of Nature, or Ghosts and Ghost-seers is a splendid collection of paranormal cases. She makes a case at the start of the book that these phenomena should not be written off as superstitious nonsense, but should be the subject of serious, logical study. Essentially, she makes a case for the scientific investigation of ghosts, spectres and all psychic phenomena.

She begins by discussing the theories of Drs Ferrier, Hibbert and Thatcher, three eminent men who had at least attempted to explain what apparitions were. They all subscribed to the belief that they had no reality, but that only certain people of a sanguine humor[6] ever saw them. Accordingly, since a sanguine person was supposed to have an excess of blood, they advocated treatment of such a person by letting their blood. Dr Ferrier cited the case of the successful treatment

---

6. See Chapter 1 and the Doctrine of Humors.

by the bleeding of someone who repeatedly saw such apparitions. Catherine Crowe admitted that she was not a medical person (although the Doctrine of Humors was an archaic and flawed medical theory), yet she did not accept that this could account for all cases. Such cases merited investigation in her opinion.

Interestingly, she suggested that mesmerism would be a suitable method of investigation to help a person to recall their experience.

Her enthusiasm for phrenology is also notable in the book. Indeed, she mentions that phrenology also can give a clue as to why some people may 'see' things:

> ... and it is not difficult to conceive that the strange, confused, and disjointed visions we are subject to on these occasions, may proceed from some parts of the brain being less at rest then the others; so that assuming phrenology to be fact, one organ is not in a state to correct the impressions of another.

As the author of *The Night Side of Nature* Catherine was much in demand when spiritualism took off mid-century. Indeed, as we saw in Chapter 8 The Coming of Spiritualism, she was invited to an early séance by Mrs Hayden. It is interesting to note that she was non-committal about whether she believed that she was actually able to communicate with the spirits.

Sadly, Catherine's reputation suffered in 1854 when she had a mental illness. The details are hard to find, so a specific medical diagnosis cannot be made. What is known is that she was found one night naked, exclaiming that spirits had made her invisible. She was admitted to a mental asylum, for there was no adequate treatment in those days. Happily, however, she did recover and she moved to London where she lived for several years before moving to Folkstone in 1871, where she passed away the following year.

DR JOSEPH RHODES BUCHANAN (1814–99)

We met Dr Buchanan in Chapter 5 Phrenology. He is also noteworthy since he was extremely active in the early investigation of psychic phenomena.

Joseph Buchanan was born in Frankfort, Kentucky, in 1814. He qualified as a doctor and became dean of the faculty of medicine at the Eclectic Medical Institute in Covington, Kentucky. Phrenology was the up-and-coming new 'science' of the mind and he immersed himself in it. Not only that, but as a practitioner of mesmerism, or hypnosis, he also combined the two into the practice that he called 'phreno-magnetism'.

In 1843 he published a neurological map showing various new faculties or organs[7] which he had discovered. He was a physiologist and he brought a

---

7. See Chapter 5 Phrenology.

clinical approach to the subject. With our hindsight, knowing that phrenology is a pseudo-science, one has to wonder at the mental mechanisms that operate to allow someone to convince themselves of the veracity of new discoveries when they were clearly based on a single false premise.

Professor Ferrier, who had developed a theory of apparitions (which Catherine Crowe alluded to in her book *The Night Side of Nature, or Ghosts and Ghost-seers*), was also a phrenologist and was working towards describing a 'centre of feeling', which could account for some people believing that they had the ability to feel beyond the five senses. Buchanan pre-empted him by describing the faculty of 'sensibility' in 1838. This faculty, he thought, when well developed, could give some the ability to sense things that other people were not aware of.

Buchanan firmly believed the views of Anton Mesmer, who had postulated that the whole universe was filled with a magnetic fluid and that the planets exerted an influence upon the human body through their effect on this invisible fluid. It was almost inevitable that he would combine his phrenological studies with mesmerism to become the founder of phreno-mesmerism.

Psychometry

Yet Buchanan's finding of the faculty of sensibility was to have an even more far-reaching consequence than phreno-mesmerism, which would of course die out when phrenology did. He began to make a serious study of people who seemed to be extremely sensitive and who could pick up on atmospheres, detect metals and minerals and tell things about people who had owned objects. In 1842 he coined the term for this ability as 'psychometry'.

His concept was an extension of Mesmer's animal magnetism. He conceived that everything that ever existed, tangible or intangible, emitted a sort of emanation and was recorded in an ethereal plane. Every object would, therefore, retain emanations from whoever had owned it. Individuals with a well-developed sensibility faculty could pick up on these emanations and give a reading of the character of a person even if they had no previous knowledge of them.

There were several people that Buchanan considered to have extreme development of the faculty. One was Bishop Leonidas Polk, who would become a general during the American Civil War. Buchanan met him in 1842 and during conversation he told him that he could detect brass just by touching it. Whenever he did he experienced a peculiar and unpleasant taste in his mouth.

This rather interesting phenomenon is not easy to explain, yet others had noted it. Indeed, Dr Justinus Kerner (1786–1862), a German physician and poet, wrote a book about a patient of his, Friederike Hauffe (1801–29), a somnambulist and possibly epileptic young girl who was apparently a gifted clairvoyant. She was the daughter of a local forester and was said to have the ability to 'read with her stomach'. Apparently she would lie down and have documents placed on her bare abdomen, before describing what was in them. In 1829 he wrote about her in a book *The Seeress of Prevorst, revelations of the human inner life and about the penetrations of the spirit world into ours.* It made her famous after her death.

Buchanan also conducted experiments on his students, some of whom seemed extremely sensitive. In an endeavour to be scientific, he gave them wrapped-up specimens of various medicines, chemicals and poisons in test tubes, which they had merely to hold and describe what was in their hands. He found that they were accurate to a far greater degree than through pure chance. Indeed, some even felt extremely ill when holding poisons like arsenic. He even found that some were so sensitive they could diagnose a patient's illness just by holding their hand.

Buchanan thought that this phenomenon heralded the beginning of a whole new science of psychometry. His belief in phreno-mesmerism led him to believe that all people would have the potential to develop psychometric ability through phreno-mesmerism, just as he believed that it was possible to enhance any of the phrenological faculties by the method:

> The past is entombed in the present, the world is its own enduring monument; and that which is true of its physical is likewise true of its mental career. The discoveries of Psychometry will enable us to explore the history of man, as those of geology enable us to explore the history of the earth. There are mental fossils for psychologists as well as mineral fossils for the geologists; and I believe that hereafter the psychologist and the geologist will go hand in hand, the one portraying the earth, its animals and its vegetation, while the other portrays the human beings who have roamed over its surface in the shadows, and the darkness of primeval barbarism. Aye, the mental telescope is now discovered which may pierce the depths of the past and bring us in full view of the grand and tragic passages of ancient history.

One eminent geologist did take up the study. Professor William Denton was inspired to test out Buchanan's theories; his interest, of course, was in minerals. In 1852 he found that his sister, Anne Denton Cridge, could hold specimens to her forehead and not only say what they were, but describe all manner of mental images that she received of them. Professor Denton went on to see how widely the faculty of sensibility was developed in the general population. He found that one in ten men had it, compared with one in four women.

Buchanan and Denton both believed firmly in psychometry.[8] Buchanan, in particular, was clearly quite genuine in thinking that mankind was on the verge of remarkable discoveries. It only needed people to grasp the method.

---

8. Psychometry is still practiced by clairvoyants and mediums and is the subject of ongoing study by parapsychologists. It may or may not have the great potential that Buchanan claimed for it.

Unfortunately, it was not the scientific world that grasped it, but the professional spiritualist mediums.

THE LONDON DIALECTICAL SOCIETY

In 1867 the London Dialectical Society was formed, consisting of gentlemen of inquiring minds. After a decade where spiritualism had rapidly expanded and mediums were giving séances or holding public meetings in cities and towns all over the country, there was seen to be a genuine need to make a scientific investigation of spiritualist phenomena. It was, after all, a highly important subject, especially in a society that saw high infant mortality and premature deaths from all manner of causes, and which saw itself as being the era of discovery and scientific advancement. In January 1869 the society resolved 'to investigate the phenomena alleged to be Spiritual Manifestations, and to report thereon'.

A committee was formed consisting of thirty-three members. Among these were representatives of the clergy, the arts, the sciences and the press: H.G. Atkinson, G. Wheatley Bennett, J.S. Bergheim, Charles Bradlaugh, G. Fenton Cameron, George Cary, E.W. Cox, Revd C. Maurice Davies, D.H. Dyte, Mrs D.H. Dyte, James Edmunds, Mrs James Edmunds, James Gannon, Grattan Geary, William B. Gower, Robert Hannah, Jenner Gale Hillier, Mrs J.G. Hillier, Henry Jeffery, H.D. Jencken, Albert Kisch, J.H. Levy, Joseph Maurice, Isaac L. Meyers, B.M. Moss, Robert Quelch, Thomas Reed, G. Russel Roberts, W.H. Sweepstone, William Volckman, Alfred Russel Wallace, Josiah Webber and Horace S. Yeomans.

The committee held fifteen meetings and received evidence from thirty-three people, who described the phenomena that they had seen or experienced. They invited evidence from sceptics and non-believers. Interestingly, they received little evidence that there was any charlatanism being practiced. They formed six sub-committees who met repeatedly, attended séances and interviewed many mediums, including D.D. Home. They published a report in 1873: *Report on Spiritualism of the Committee of the London Dialectical Society together with the evidence, oral and written and a selection of the correspondence.*

Their conclusion was that the phenomena that they had considered – including levitation, apparition of spirit hands, playing of instruments by unseen aid, holding of red-hot coals without injury, messages from rapping, automatic writing, slate writing, the appearance of drawings, the appearance of flowers, elongation of the body and the appearance of faces in crystals – were genuine and that they detected no evidence of imposture, delusion or fraudulence. They suggested that it all was worthy of further scientific investigation.

Alfred Russel Wallace, the great scientist who developed theories on evolution, was a staunch supporter of spiritualism. He wrote in his book *On Miracles and Modern Spiritualism* in 1875, that of the thirty-three members only eight of them believed in the phenomena at the start of their investigation. During the course of the investigation twelve sceptics became convinced of the reality of the phenomena and at least three actually became spiritualists.

The report was certainly a great coup for the cause of spiritualism, despite the fact that much of the press were critical of the findings. The thing was that an eminent body of learned men and women had found in its favour.

THE GHOST CLUB

In 1855 several fellows at Trinity College, Cambridge, met to discuss the nature of ghostly phenomena. It was an informal group which actually formed into a club in London in 1862. It attracted many eminent Victorians, including the celebrated writer Charles Dickens. It is said to be the oldest such club in the world, the purpose of which was to investigate all ghostly and psychic phenomena, including contacts with the spirit world that were an integral part of the spiritualist movement.

In 1862 the Ghost Club, as it was know, investigated the Davenport brothers, whom we met briefly in Chapter 8 The Coming of Spiritualism, and will meet again in Chapter 14 The Egyptian Hall. These brothers performed in halls all over the country, using a special spirit cabinet in which they were tied, and from which all manner of ghostly phenomena were said to emerge. The Ghost Club did not seem to discover anything amiss.

It is not clear how sympathetic the Ghost Club was to mediums in its first incarnation, for it temporarily dissolved in 1870 upon the death of Charles Dickens. Dickens was always intrigued by the possibility of spirits, but was sceptical. It would arise again, however, in 1882 when it was 'refounded' by the Reverend Stainton Moses, who by then was famous for his skills as a medium, and Alfred Alaric Watts. From then on it seemed to be a club for individuals who were avid believers in the spirit world.

This is not to say, however, that its members were excessively credulous, since there were many eminent scientists and professional men in its ranks. Professor Sir William Crookes and Sir Oliver Lodge were active members, as was Sir Arthur Conan Doyle in later years.

THE PSYCHOLOGICAL SOCIETY

In April 1875 the Psychological Society was formed. It was founded by Edward William Cox (1809–79), who had been on the investigating committee of the London Dialectical Society. He was a barrister and enjoyed the title of sergeant, which was an order of the English Bar that had been in existence since the days of King Henry II until it was abolished in 1921. Other founding members included the Reverend William Stainton Moses, Walter H. Coffin and C.C. Massey. The aim of the society was to investigate what they described as 'psychical science' or, quite loosely, psychology.

Sergeant Cox took the view that psychic phenomena were real, but they weren't the work of spirits or entities. He felt sure that they could be explained in terms of science. He himself conducted much research into the matter, together with Sir William Crookes. However, although the aims of the society were laudable, they did not seem to have sufficient scientific expertise to conduct the research and it closed when Cox died in 1879. Nevertheless, it had sparked off a desire to investigate the phenomena in a co-ordinated and scientific manner.

THE SOCIETY FOR PSYCHICAL RESEARCH

In 1882, the first really systematic study of spiritualism and psychic phenomena began when the Society for Psychical Research (SPR) was founded in London by the philosopher Henry Sedgwick. His co-founders were the physicists Sir Oliver Lodge, Sir William Barrett and Sir William Crookes, and the philosophers Frederick W.H. Myers and Edmund Gurney. The Reverend William Stainton Moses was also a prominent early member, but he, along with several other confirmed spiritualists, left soon after when they disagreed with the direction that the society was taking regarding its investigations.

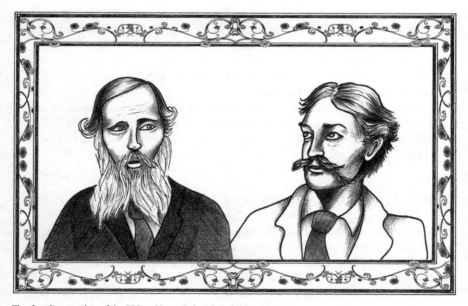

Two founding members of the SPR – Henry Sedgwick and Edmund Gurney.

The society decided shortly after it was formed that it needed to be systematic in its approach to the many phenomena that came under its aegis. Accordingly, it formed five areas of investigation, each with its leading researcher and its own committee. These were:

The possibility that one mind may influence another

The study of all hypnotic phenomena

The investigation of Reichenbach's Odic Force and his supposition that sensitive individual's could pick up on its emanations

The investigation of any apparitions present at the time of death, hauntings and ghostly phenomena

The investigation of the physical phenomena that were associated with spiritualism

In 1885, following a meeting between Sedgwick and the psychologist William James, a sister organisation came into being with the founding of the American Society for Psychical Research. Soon investigations into all of these areas were underway on both sides of the Atlantic. They are still in progress today.

A CASE OF CREDULITY

Edmund Gurney (1847–88) was a psychologist who studied medicine, although he never qualified as a doctor. Instead he devoted himself to 'psychical science' research. Between 1874 and 1878 he had worked with several professional mediums, but was unconvinced with the results that they obtained. It was for this reason that he felt the need for a proper organisation to be formed, thus he became the honorary secretary of the Society for Psychical Research. He was especially interested in the possibility of telepathy and thought that hypnosis was a way that it could be demonstrated.

Between 1883 and 1888 Gurney worked with George Albert Smith (1864–1959), a professional hypnotist, psychic and pioneer in cinema. Smith was one half of a mind reading act, along with Douglas Blackburn. He claimed that the act was a genuine demonstration of telepathic communication, which was accepted as the truth by the society. He then joined and became private secretary to Edmund Gurney.

The experiments that were performed were done using Smith as the hypnotist. The results seemed to offer incredibly compelling evidence that telepathy was a real phenomenon that could be tapped into during the hypnotic state. Gurney established a considerable reputation as a researcher on the basis of the results and wrote his magnum opus, *Phantasms of the Living*, which was published in 1886. Unfortunately, in 1888 he apparently discovered that Smith may have been using his show business skills to bias or even create the results.

Sadly, Gurney died in Brighton soon after as the result of a chloroform overdose. It is strongly suspected that he could have committed suicide. As for

Smith, he continued to work at the society as secretary to Frederick W.H. Myers. He even co-authored a paper in the society's journal on thought transference. He left the society in 1892.

THE FIRST PRESIDENT

Henry Sidgwick (1838–1900) was the first president of the Society for Psychical Research. He was a philosopher, economist and a campaigner for higher education for women. Indeed, it was largely through his work that Newnham College, Cambridge, was founded.

He was born in Skipton in Yorkshire, the son of a clergyman. He was educated at Trinity College, Cambridge, as was Edmund Gurney. In due course he became a fellow of the college, but resigned in 1869 since he felt that he could not in all conscience claim to be a member of the Church of England. At that time it was a pre-requisite for the fellowship. In 1883 he became professor of philosophy and two years after that, when the religious test was dropped, he was again elected to the fellowship. This position he took did not mean that he was an atheist. Indeed, he considered himself to be a believer in something, yet it was not the doctrine of the Orthodox Church.

In 1876 he had married Eleanor Balfour (1845–1936) who was one of the first women to enter Newnham College. She eventually became vice-principal and then principal. Together, she and her husband were prominent researchers within the society. She followed him and became president herself in 1908, then president of honour in 1932.

They were very interested in telepathy and conducted extensive experiments between 1889 and 1891, using George Smith as the hypnotist. The experiments consisted of a 'receiver volunteer' being hypnotised and then separated from another 'projecting volunteer' by a screen. The projecting volunteer would try to project images or numbers to the receiver. It is notable that George Smith also acted as both a receiver and as a projector in experiments.

The results were found to be significantly better than chance and their conclusion was that there seemed to be evidence for thought transference.

SYMPATHETIC MEMBERS

Although many of the early investigators were very sceptical, others were at best sympathetic and at times over-credulous.

Frederic William Henry Myers (1843–1901) was a poet and scholar. He became interested in spiritualism in 1873. It was at this time that he fell in love with his married cousin. Tragically, her husband was committed to a mental asylum and she drowned herself. Although he later married, he never stopped loving his cousin, Annie Marshall, and fervently hoped that he would communicate with her or meet her again in another life. He was perhaps not as objective as was required to be an effective researcher, and it seems that on several occasions he was duped by some fraudulent mediums. A posthumous work entitled *Human Personality and its Survival of Bodily Death* was published in 1903.

Sir Oliver Lodge (1851–1940) was a physicist who was deeply involved with communication by wireless telegraphy, or early radio. He had been interested in psychic phenomena and was a member of the Ghost Club in the 1880s. His membership of the Society of Psychical Research was very welcome, since he was such a scientist of note. He was to become president of the society from 1901 to 1903. If anyone could bring objectivity to the study of such phenomena it was surely he. Yet he, too, was ready to be convinced. When he witnessed some of the medium Eusapia Palladino's materialisations he declared that he was satisfied that he knew of no agency that could be responsible for her manifestations.

The First World War would later hugely boost interest in spiritualism as millions of bereaved families sought solace after the loss of a whole generation of its youth. Sir Oliver Lodge lost his son, Raymond, in the conflict, and from 1915 he visited many mediums in the hope of receiving communications from him. He wrote extensively about this and his book *Raymond, or Life and Death* became a bestseller after it was published in 1916.

Sir William Crookes (1832–1919) was a chemist and physicist, whose name is embedded in the history of physics. He was a pioneer in spectroscopy and among other things he invented the Crookes tube, an electrical discharge tube used for studying cathode rays.

From the late 1860s he developed an interest in spiritualism and in 1870 expressed the opinion that science should be actively studying psychic phenomena. It is likely that his interest was sparked off by the death of his brother in 1861 from yellow fever while he was working abroad. He did bring a scientific approach to his study of these phenomena, stipulating that he had to be able to control the experiment:

> It must be at my own house, and my own selection of friends and spectators, under my own conditions, and I may do whatever I like as regards apparatus.

Nevertheless, he may not have realised just how ingenious people can be. Magicians make their living by making people see and believe that they are witnessing the impossible before their very eyes; they do it as illusion. Fraudulent mediums did it and claimed it as reality.

Among the mediums that Crookes watched under his controlled conditions were Kate Fox, Florence Cook and D.D. Home. He failed to find any evidence of fraudulence by them or other mediums. The phenomena that he saw covered the whole range of levitation, body elongation, spirit writing and materialisations. He declared that he could not account for them and that they had to be happening through some unknowable outside agency.

Like Sir Oliver Lodge, he was a welcome member of the Society for Psychical Research because of his scientific pedigree. His conclusions, on the other hand, did not sit well with those of his scientific peers. Indeed, there was even discussion about whether he should have his fellowship of the Royal Society revoked.

We cannot conclude this section without mentioning Professor Alfred Russel Wallace. He was an explorer, geographer, naturalist and biologist who, independently from Darwin, came up with a theory of evolution. He was interested in all manner of subjects and in a way epitomised the Victorian open-minded scientist. He was a believer in phrenology and in spiritualism, which did not sit well with other scientists who accepted his ideas on evolution. His outré views were considered paradoxical, to say the least.

It was his defence of several mediums who were alleged to have committed fraud that angered so many of his colleagues. Yet despite their ire he held true to himself and continued to hold faith in them and in the reality of at least some of the psychic phenomena that mediums produced.

THE CHANGING FACE OF SPIRITUALISM

The Society for Psychical Research did have a major impact on the activities of many mediums. The materialisations that had been so common in the 1870s became less common, since so many mediums had been exposed. Many, therefore, shifted the emphasis of their séances to the production of spirit writing. Then, in 1886, a major blow to spirit writing was levelled when a magician set about a major exposure.

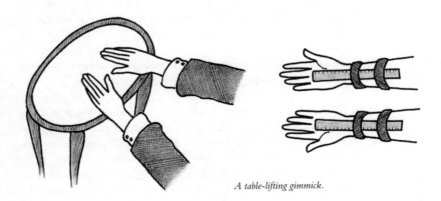

A table-lifting gimmick.

S.T. Davey, an amateur magician, studied the spirit writing of mediums and applied his knowledge of conjuring to see how he could duplicate their work. He was soon able to do so very competently and so, together with Richard Hodgson, his manager, he set up as a medium. Over the course of twenty séances he produced every type of spirit writing, caused objects to levitate, performed thought reading and materialised spirit forms. He gathered a reputation and then revealed himself a magician, before a paper appeared outlining everything in the proceedings of the Society of Psychical Research.

Alfred Russel Wallace responded to this and suggested that not all he claimed could be ascribed to conjuring, and suggested that he may in fact have been a medium, unknown to himself. This rather odd suggestion was an argument that spiritualists often used in defence of mediums who had been caught out. It was suggested that the spirits could not always produce the phenomena and that sometimes they needed physical help. The medium was not, therefore, guilty of deliberate falsification, but was working under spirit control.

The furore that followed this resulted in many spiritualists leaving the society.

12

THEOSOPHY

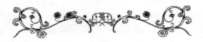

Theosophy, in its abstract meaning, is Divine Wisdom, or the aggregate of the knowledge and wisdom that underlie the Universe – the homogeneity of eternal GOOD; and in its concrete sense it is the sum total of the same as allotted to man by nature, on this earth, and no more.

The Key to Theosophy, 1889
H.P. Blavatsky

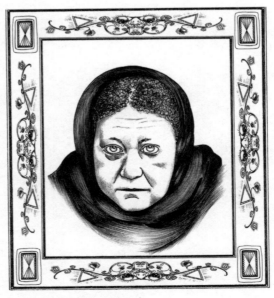

Madame Helena Petrovna Blavatsky.

Spiritualism was thriving in the Victorian era, but the continued attacks on the credibility of mediums and the sporadic exposure of undoubted fraudulent ones had begun to impinge upon its reputation. Nonetheless, it had catered for a need in people that did not seem to be met by orthodox religions. Also, as the British Empire expanded people became aware that there were many other religions on offer and the inevitable question arose: how can all religions purport to be the one that holds the truth? Some of these other religions, like Hinduism, Buddhism and Sikhism, for example, which were widely practiced in India and the countries to the East, seemed very exotic and very attractive. They had an appealing mystery to them. Could there be something like spiritualism that was not so rooted in Western thought? Could there be some way of tapping into the other religions and philosophies in a way that made them comprehensible to the Western mind?

The answer was an emphatic 'yes'. And the person who was going to bring this new way of thinking, which she would call 'theosophy', was a spiritualist who would soon become famous across the world as Madame Blavatsky.

THEOSOPHY

In the late 1870s, Madame Helena Petrovna Blavatsky (1831–91) co-founded the Theosophical Society with Colonel Harry Steel Olcott in Madras, India. The term 'theosophy' comes from the Greek words *theos*, meaning 'god', and *sophia*, meaning 'wisdom'. According to the movement's teachings, all religions stem from a common root of ancient wisdom, which can be discerned from the common myths and symbols which abound, and a study of these will lead to truth and spiritual unity.

Within this framework man is conceived of as a spiritual being, and there are seven spheres of consciousness, or seven subtle bodies. The physical body is the lowest of these and since this is the main one that we perceive and are aware of, we tend to pay it most attention. The higher ones are harder to feel or be aware of, which explains why most people have such difficulty with their spiritual lives. At least that is the idea.

A central tenet of theosophy is the concept of karma-governed reincarnation. That is, the belief that we live through a succession of lives, each one of which has a purpose of teaching us a basic principle. Karma is essentially a principle whereby one reaps what one sews. Therefore, if one makes a bad mistake or transgresses from good action, the universe will repay you in kind. Your life will not learn the lesson and you may be doomed to another incarnation until you learn the lessons that your individual soul needs to learn.

This was an amazingly successful movement which offered a mid-way between magic and religion. The theosophists talked about the ancient wisdom of the Tibetans and explained how such knowledge could be given to the enlightened Western mind.

MADAME BLAVATSKY

A co-founder of the movement, Helena Petrovna Blavatsky was born into the noble German family of von Hahn. Her father was a colonel in the army and her mother was a successful author.

Helena's life was quite remarkable. She was from an early age a woman driven by change and she was comelled to travel, to wander and to search. In particular she felt a desire to search for understanding and enlightenment, and this search would take her across the world, seeking out the wisdom of the ancients.

At the age of 17 she married the vice-governor of Erivan in Armenia. He was a man much older than she and according to her the marriage was never consummated. Indeed, she claimed to have remained a virgin all of her life. After a miserable three months she ran away, riding on horseback to her grandfather's home across the mountains. He in turn decided that she should stay with her father so sent her to Odessa, where he arranged for her father to collect her. However, when he arrived, she had already left and made for Turkey instead.

She spent the next ten years travelling around Europe and the East. In 1858 she went to Russia as a spiritualist and began to build a reputation as a medium. Over the next dozen years she consolidated that reputation, her wanderlust taking her all over the world including, by her own account, a considerable stay with advanced masters in Tibet. She said that these masters, or 'mahatmas', taught her many of the mysteries that she proposed to teach to others. It is known that for a while she studied with the medium D.D. Home. Finally, she moved to America and took up American citizenship.

It was there that she gave up her spiritualist roots. She met Colonel Harry Steel Olcott and together they formulated the concepts of theosophy. In 1875 they formed the Theosophical Society in New York. Its original purpose was to foster the study of occultism and esoteric knowledge. Yet again, India drew her, since it was for her the source of the ancient wisdom that she desired. In 1878 they moved the headquarters of the movement to Madras.

Theosophy proved to be very popular in India and soon people were travelling there from all over the world to learn about this new movement.

It had three main objectives:

To become a nucleus for universal brotherhood regardless of race, class or creed
To encourage study of all sciences, religions and philosophies
To study and investigate the many unexplained laws of nature and the dormant powers in humans

There was much that was attractive in this movement that was quite distinct from spiritualism, yet which also had similarities. Its main difference, of course, revolved around the belief in reincarnation, since it implied that although an individual lived through a series of separate lives, each was distinct. Spiritualism, on the other hand, suggested that each life was unique and that it survived death but then remained in the spirit world as that unique spirit.

THE MAHATMAS

These individuals that Madame Blavatsky claimed to have studied under were supposedly people who had reached an advanced state of enlightenment through leading an aesthetic life. They could travel outside of their bodies by astral projection, use telepathy over any distance and could observe people anywhere by the mere exercise of their will. More than that, they could cause objects to be transported from one place to another, passing through walls, locked doors or safes. Indeed, should a mahatma will it, anything was possible. Madame Blavatsky claimed to be a 'chela', or an apprentice, to them.

She wrote extensively about theosophy, notably in her 1877 book *Isis Unveiled* (which she claimed the goddess Isis herself actually imparted to her) and her 1888 magnum opus *The Secret Doctrine*. She taught that the mahatmas were not mere wizards, but were guides whose aim was to teach humanity and to help it evolve as part of an overall cosmic process.

In 1886 she travelled to Belgium where she stayed for a year before finally moving to London, where she would live out the rest of her life until her death in 1891.

PSYCHIC CORRESPONDENCE

Word travelled fast about the many wonderful phenomena that were being witnessed in India and people flocked to learn more, to witness these wonders and to investigate them for veracity.

Many of these phenomena were of the same order as the rappings, materialisations and transportations that were practiced by the spiritualist mediums in their séance parlours across Britain and America.

Then, in 1881, a mysterious 'correspondence', which has come to be known as the Mahatma Letters, took place between Madame Blavatsky and the English medium William Eglinton. Eglinton had been visiting interested spiritualists in Calcutta and had gained some celebrity following articles about his séances in the *Indian Mirror* newspaper.

While there he amazed people by getting his spirit control, Ernest, to take handwritten letters from Calcutta to England and back again in a matter of minutes. The returned letters had replies from the writer's friends in England. Following this he sent Ernest to Tothill Fields Prison in Westminster, London, to bring a ring belonging to Mrs Susie Fletcher, a medium who had been sentenced to twelve months' hard labour for obtaining property from another woman by undue influence. The provenance of the ring was 'proven' by the appearance of a subsequent letter in her handwriting, saying that she had sent the letter.

In 1882 Eglinton sailed home from India and whilst on the ship claimed to have been contacted by Koot Hoomi, a mahatma. He wrote a letter and it was immediately transported to a room in Bombay in which Madame Blavatsky was sitting with friends. The letter was addressed to a Mrs Gordon. Madame Blavatsky jotted some notes on a visiting card, wrapped that in the letter and sent it on by psychic post to Calcutta, where it materialised at another meeting in a room attended by Mr and Mrs Gordon and Colonel Harry Steel Olcott.

Both Blavatsky and Eglinton claimed that they had never met.

THE SOCIETY FOR PSYCHICAL RESEARCH

Inevitably, the SPR became interested in the comings and goings (literally) of the Theosophical Society and sent an investigator, Richard Hodgson, to India in 1884. This followed a series of letters that were published in the *Madras Christian College Magazine*, purportedly written by Madame Blavatsky to a French couple, Alexis and Emma Coulomb. This couple had been members of the society, but had been expelled. The essence of the letters was that many of the psychic phenomena that had been reported were simply fakes.

By this time Madame Blavatsky and Colonel Olcott had left for England, so Hodgson had a pretty free hand in his investigation. Emma Coulomb showed him the letters and he was also able to examine rooms where phenomena were said to have occurred. He found fresh plasterwork that concealed channels or openings and a sliding panel. His report, which ran to over 200 pages, supported the Coulombs and badly dented Madame Blavatsky's reputation. He said that she was one of the most gifted, ingenious and interesting imposters in history.

THEOSOPHY AFTER BLAVATSKY

When Madame Blavatsky died the movement fragmented. There were disputes about its direction and philosophy, but if anything it seems that the disputes were about power. That said, the Theosophical Society is still very active today, with chapters in many countries including India, Britain and the United States. No longer are the psychic phenomena a part of their practice, it is a movement that seeks knowledge and understanding of life, basically following the precepts that Blavatsky and Olcott originally formulated.

PART THREE

MAGICIANS

13

FROM ANCIENT EGYPT TO ENGLISH MUSIC HALLS

But whereas the magic of every other nation of the ancient East was directed entirely against the powers of darkness … the Egyptians aimed at being able to command their gods to work for them, and to compel them to appear at their desire.

Egyptian Magic, 1899
E.A. Wallis Budge

The origin of the word 'magic' is obscure. Some aver that it is derived from the Greek *mageia* and the Latin *magia*, yet others suggest that it comes from words that were once spoken by the ancients. A cuneiform tablet excavated at Behistan is said to have a character for the word *mugh*, meaning 'fire-worshipper'. And in Babylon the word *mag* meant 'priest'. It is from this that the society of the *Magi*, the wise men, is said to have developed.

The practice of conjuring or the art of illusion, as opposed to the practice of actual magic, is very ancient. Anthropologists tell us that in early tribal societies medicine men, shamans and witch-doctors fulfilled a highly important position. They were the link between earthly life and the gods, they were the suppliers of medicine, gave hope of divine help and favour, and gave protection from the evil spirits who seemed to be ever ready to possess people or take their souls. Through ritual, trances and the use of wands, bones, knucklebones and possibly animal sacrifice, they were the possessors of power and influence.

Yet when the rituals, dances and incantations failed to work it seems that the medicine men would resort to tricks. By causing things to vanish or disappear, change form through well-executed sleight of hand, or through the use of some special magical apparatus they could demonstrate their skill.

This amalgamation of medicine, the occult and conjuring in one person is fascinating, for it suggests that the three areas that we are considering throughout this book do have an archaic origin. It implies that they were all at one time part and parcel of the same endeavour, which was to emphasise to others that the medicine man did have extra-special power. Ironically, as we shall see in this third part of the book, it was the modern-day magician, the entertainer, who started to shed light on the mountebanks and fraudulent mediums who prayed upon the credulous in the Victorian era.

ANCIENT EGYPT

The first recorded reference to magic is found in the *Westcar Papyrus* of 1500 BC, now housed in the Ägyptisches Museum in Berlin. It recounts the performance of the magician Tchatcha-em-ank, also known by the shorter name of Dedi, at the court of King Khufu, the pharaoh who built the Great Pyramid at Giza.

The Westcar Papyrus is named after Henry Westcar, a collector of Egyptian antiquities, who acquired it in 1824. It was sold to the German Egyptologist Richard Lepsius on a visit to England in 1838. When he died it was donated to the Ägyptisches Museum in Berlin, where it is preserved under low-light conditions.

The papyrus is incomplete, having lost its beginning and end, yet it gives a fascinating insight into the ancient Egyptian belief in magic. It recounts several tales (although we do not know how many it originally contained) told to King Khufu (also known as Cheops) by his sons.

Only a few lines remain of the first story, which is about a magician whose name is lost in the missing passages. It is set during the reign of King Djoser, the pharaoh of the third dynasty who built the famous Step Pyramid, around 2500 BC.

The second story is also fragmentary and is about a priest of Ptah called Weba-aner during the reign of King Nebka, who ruled before Djoser. He is said to have turned a wax model of a crocodile into a real 12ft monster which seized and devoured Weba-aner's wife's lover and devoured him, before being transformed back into a model of wax.

The third is set during the reign of King Sneferu of the fourth dynasty and concerns Jajamanekh, another priest of Ptah, who recovered a piece of turquoise jewellery dropped by a lady in a lake. By magic he parted the waters and moved one half on top of the other so that the jewellery could be retrieved. Dr E.A. Wallis Budge, who had been the Keeper of Egyptian and Assyrian Antiquities at the British Museum, wrote in his book *Egyptian Magic* that this predated Moses' parting of the Red Sea by centuries.

The fourth story was told by Prince Dedefhra, who would become pharaoh after Khufu. It is interesting because it tells of our magician Tchatcha-em-ank, or Dedi, who was a performer rather than a priest.

According to the Westcar Papyrus, Prince Dedefhra had been sceptical of his brothers' tales of the magician-priests and told his father that he knew of a living magician rather than one from the old days, and that this wonder-worker was already 110 years old and lived not far away. He had a prodigious appetite and every day ate a shoulder of beef, 500 loaves and drank 100 jugs of beer. King Khufu ordered that the magician should be invited to the court to perform for him. When he arrived he was offered a condemned prisoner in order to perform a decapitation trick. The magician declined, since he said that it was not for him to take a human life. Instead, in turn he decapitated and restored to life a goose, a pelican and an ox.

THE PROPHET DANIEL AND THE HUNGRY IDOL

In the Biblical Apocrypha the tale is told of the prophet Daniel who lived during the reign of the Persian King Cyrus, who conquered the Babylonians. Daniel was a companion and friend of his.

The Babylonians worshiped an idol called Bel, which was kept in a sealed shrine. King Cyrus informed Daniel that Bel was a great god, because every day he consumed 12 bushels of flour, 40 sheep and 50 gallons of wine. Cyrus was mightily impressed by this, but less than impressed by Daniel who refused to bow before the idol. In reply Daniel said that the idol was simply a statue, and not a true god. Cyrus was angered and summoned the priests of Bel, demanding that they prove who consumed the daily feast. If they could show that Bel consumed the provisions then Daniel would die for blasphemy against the god. If they did not then they would die.

There were seventy priests of Bel together with their families. They accepted the challenge and offered that the king should himself lay the provisions in the shrine after they had gone. So this Cyrus did, but before sealing the door to the shrine Daniel sprinkled ash over the floor.

The next day the provisions had all gone and Cyrus imagined that Bel had consumed everything. Then Daniel showed him the footprints in the ash on the floor, evidence that the priests and their families had entered the shrine through a secret door under the altar.

Interestingly, this subterfuge seems to have been used by Sir Arthur Conan Doyle in the Sherlock Holmes short story *The Adventure of the Golden Pince-Nez*. Conan Doyle tells the story in his own inimitable magical way of how the great detective discovers a secret room by surreptitiously dropping a fine patina of cigarette ash over a floor as he walks back and forth.

THE CUPS AND BALLS

A wall mural dating from 2000 BC, from the tomb of Baqet III at Beni Hasan, a small village not far from Cairo, is said to depict a conjuror performing what is regarded as one of the oldest tricks in the world, the famed cups and balls. This depiction has been cited in many books on the history of magic, although it has to be admitted that contemporary historians of performing magic are doubtful that it actually shows the trick being performed. Rather, they suggest it is a portrayal of bakers at work. This may be true, yet there is still a case to be made for the conjuring trick, since other paintings in the same tomb very clearly show jugglers and acrobats at work.

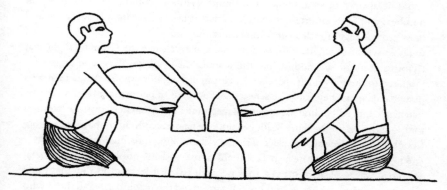

The cups and balls at Beni Hasan in ancient Egypt.

Whether this picture shows the magic trick or not is probably never going to be categorically proven one way or the other. Nevertheless, we know that the trick which involves the seeming disappearance of balls from under one cup and their reappearance under another has been performed for centuries. Performers in ancient Rome performed this effect, which they referred to as the *acetabuli et calculi*. This is Latin for 'vinegar cups and stones'.

In the fifteenth century the artist Hieronymus Bosch (1450–1516) painted *The Conjuror* in about 1475, showing a magician performing the trick while an accomplice cuts the purse off the belt of a spectator. Clearly, it refers to the lowly and disreputable status of conjurors who were bracketed along with cut-purses and other thieves.

Another artist, Pieter Breugel the Elder, also depicted a conjuror performing the cups and balls trick in his painting *Saint Jacques and the Magician Hermogenes* in 1565. This fascinating picture shows the saint confronted by a conjuror and a number of jugglers performing all manner of incredible tricks aided by their diabolical 'familiars'.

The trick demands a degree of sleight of hand or manual dexterity and has been popular with magicians throughout the ages. The modern-day British magician Paul Daniels has taken it to a new level, performing it with only one cup. He has made it his signature trick.

It has even gained royal approval, in that HRH Prince Charles performed the trick at his audition to become a member of the famous Magic Circle.

THE RISE OF THE MOUNTEBANKS

In medieval days streets and market squares were places where business was conducted. That was where performing troupes of players, jugglers and acrobats could be assured of an audience. Undoubtedly there would have been safety in numbers and such entertainers would arrive at taverns, set up a crude stage and draw crowds eager for diversion and entertainment.

Those were not safe days for performers, however, since the Church taught that all forms of magic was nothing but the work of the devil. For those conjurors who promised to show wonders that they had brought back from strange lands, there was potential danger. They could be arrested and accused of performing black magic or witchcraft. Indeed, because so many rural magistrates had brought so many performers to trial and even imposed the death penalty, one far-sighted Kentish magistrate wrote a book to show that these displays of magic were nothing more than trickery.

The magistrate's name was Reginald Scott and his book *The Discoverie of Witchcraft* was published in 1584. In it he went to great length to show that there was a large difference between those who practiced the magical arts and those who sought merely to entertain. He explained and showed by means of illustrations how many tricks were done. This included the so-called 'decollation of John Baptist', whereby a decapitated yet animated head lay on a salver alongside the body of a man. This was actually one of the 'diabolical tricks' that was illustrated in Pieter Breugal the Elder's painting *Saint Jacques and the Magician Hermogenes*, mentioned above. Scott's book was effectively the first textbook on conjuring.

Seemingly the book had some effect in educating magistrates about harmless conjurors, since arrests and prosecutions lessened. They did not completely stop, of course, and many a performer was forced to reveal his secrets to prevent punishment by over-zealous magistrates who still believed that their mysteries were the work of the devil.

One such person who was not convinced by the book was none other than King James I. He authorised a new version of the Bible (the King James Bible) and prided himself on his own scholarship. In 1604 he wrote a treatise entitled *A Counterblaste to Tobacco*, warning people about the dangers of smoking. Nonetheless, he was blinkered wherever a mention was made about witchcraft. He ordered that all copies of Scott's book that could be obtained should be burned by the public executioner.

Paradoxically, King James was actually rather fond of performed magic and was entertained on several occasions by William Vincent, a magician who wrote a treatise *Hocus Pocus junior, the Anatomy of Legerdemain* in 1634. He famously used the words *Hocus pocus, tontus, talontus, vade celeriter jubeo* in order to misdirect his audience from his sleight of hand.

Those solitary performers who were less celebrated than Vincent often used their shows to attract crowds so that they could then sell elixirs or nostrums of some sort or another, claiming all sorts of extravagant results. Many claimed to be physicians, surgeons or dentists and they plied their trade with vigour. Hair-restorers, tooth-whitening remedies, tooth-growing potions and aphrodisiacs made of weird and wonderful ingredients would have been sold and eagerly purchased. And, of course, the seller would have been long gone before the results were found to be useless.

Such folk were declared mountebanks, because they would 'mount a bench' and proclaim their skills.

MAGICIANS AT THE FAIRS

Street entertainers in the sixteenth and seventeenth centuries tended to carry their props around with them. Magicians were often depicted in paintings wearing leather aprons with a large pocket in front from which they could remove their tricks. This also doubled as a convenient place to deftly drop things into when they needed to make objects disappear. In France such a magician's apron was called a *gibecière*.

Some magicians also wore a 'budget', a small pouch that hung from a belt. This may well have been the origin for the term 'bag of tricks'.

Performing tricks in the round, with spectators able to see what was going on from all angles, would limit the type of tricks that could be performed. Having a transportable bench that one could hop up on and position close to a wall to limit the view of what went on 'behind the scenes' became increasingly common. And with this mini-stage, or bench, the magicians gradually made their acts more sophisticated. Doing away with the apron, they wore more dandified clothes to make them seem possessed of greater wealth and power, all of which added to the sense of illusion. Others would wear voluminous gowns or cloaks evocative of the mysterious lands of the East, which they would claim to have visited and brought back magical secrets from. Many adopted grand and extravagant-sounding names, and claimed fictitious titles or relationships to equally fictitious kings or emperors.

In the eighteenth century magicians would incorporate small conjuror's tables complete with table cover and banner proclaiming their name. Most importantly, they would also have a pocket, or *servante*, hanging down the back of the table into which things would disappear, or things like birds, rabbits or cakes could be lifted from underneath and thus magically produced.

One of the most celebrated itinerant magicians of the early eighteenth century was Isaac Fawkes, who performed under the name of Fawkes or sometimes just Faux. Fairgoers would be attracted in droves to see 'Faux's dexterity of hand'.

He regularly had a booth at Bartholomew Fair and also at Southwark Fair. In 1720 he is recorded as having his own theatre room at the Cock and Half Moon Tavern. His signature trick was the 'hen bag', now commonly known and performed as the 'egg bag'; a simple cloth bag which can be turned inside out, yet from which the conjuror can produce a dozen or so eggs.[9]

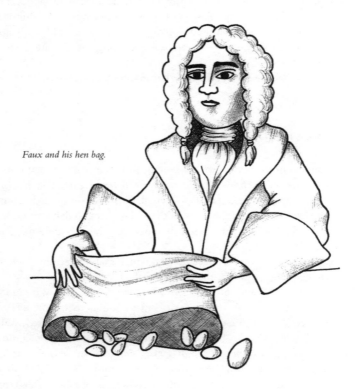

Faux and his hen bag.

Significantly, Fawkes was one of the first magicians to feature an automaton in his show. This was called the 'Temple of the Arts' and involved mechanical battleships and marching soldiers on the Rock of Gibraltar. In this he laid the foundations for some of the great stage illusionists who would come after him, notably Robert-Houdin and John Nevil Maskelyne, whom we shall meet later in the book.

---

9. A modification of this is one of the author's favourite tricks, which he performed at his long-suffering children's parties as Marcel Cookie! In this the egg bag is shaped like a chef's hat, which also has the undetectable secret pocket for the production of the egg.

Fawkes became something of a sensation in his day and was even visited in the Haymarket in 1722 by Prince George, later to become King George II. Apparently, the prince was highly satisfied and amazed by the performance.

The eighteenth century also saw a number of performing families coming to prominence. They were effectively circus troupes, each of whom would specialise in a certain type of act. The Gyngells were such a family, who regularly performed in London and on tour between 1788 and 1833.

Mr Gyngell was a card specialist, able to perform countless card sleights and flourishes; his wife sang; their eldest son, Joseph, was a juggler; the middle son, Horatio, danced and performed acrobatics; while George, the youngest, was a fire-eater and tight-rope artist.

COMING IN FROM THE COLD

The Victorian era saw a shift in entertainment from fairs to the yards of taverns. Many enterprising proprietors of inns and public houses made rooms available for various types of entertainers. These became the saloon bars. They varied in quality, according to the location and clientele of the establishment, but gradually they became regular venues for travelling entertainers of all types. By the mid-nineteenth century purpose-built music halls then started to appear.

The first one was the Canterbury Hall in Lambeth in London, which opened its doors in 1852. It was built on the site of an old skittle alley. Customers paid for their drinks and received free entertainment. So successful was the Canterbury Hall that its owner, Charles Morton, rebuilt it in 1854 with a large stage and room for 1,500 people. This was the blueprint. Soon, music halls sprang up in large towns and cities all over the country. This is what Charles Dickens Jr, son of the great Victorian novelist, had to say about the music halls in his book *Dickens's Dictionary of London 1879*:

> The music hall, as it is at present understood, was started many years ago at the Canterbury Hall over the water. The entertainments proving popular, the example was speedily followed in every quarter of the town. The performance in no way differs, except in magnitude, from those which are to be seen in every town of any importance throughout the country. Ballet, gymnastics, and so-called comic-singing, form the staple of the bill of fare, but nothing comes foreign to the music hall proprietor. Performing animals, winners of walking matches, successful scullers, shipwrecked sailors, swimmers of the Channel, conjurors, ventriloquists, tight-rope dancers, campanologists, clog-dancers, sword-swallowers, velocipedists, champion skaters, imitators, marionettes, decanter equilibrists, champion shots, 'living models of marble gems,' 'statue marvels,' 'fire princes,' 'mysterious youths,' 'spiral bicycle ascensionists,' flying children, empresses of the air, kings of the wire, 'vital sparks,' 'Mexican boneless wonders,' 'white-eyed musical Kaffirs,' strong-jawed

ladies, cannon-ball performers, illuminated fountains, and that remarkable musical eccentricity the orchestra militaire, all have had their turn on the music hall stage.

He went on to list the various London music halls. In his *Dickens's Dictionary of London 1888* he mentions that the Coburg had been converted into a music hall on 'temperance' principles.

Among all of the weird and wonderful acts, magicians were much in demand. They had developed into a recognisable entertainment profession, some would say into the very backbone of the Victorian music halls, and many of them were to become huge stars.

14

THE EGYPTIAN HALL

PICCADILLY (Map 6) – This building has for some years been successfully
occupied by Messrs Maskelyne & Cooke's Entertainment. NEAREST *Ry Stn.*,
St James-pk; *Omnibus Rtes.*, Piccadilly and Regent st; *Cab Rank*, Albany

Dickens's Dictionary of London 1888

Charles Dickens Jr

In 1812 a most remarkable building was erected in London's Piccadilly. It was
a tall, exotic-looking building which was almost pylon-shaped with papyrus
columns flanking its doors and with great statues of the Egyptian gods Isis and
Osiris on either side of a first-floor window. Carved ankhs and a crocodile
enhanced its façade. The design was based on that of an Egyptian
temple and eventually it became known as the Egyptian
Hall. In time it would become known as the
Home of Mystery.

Yet it did not start out with that name.
It was originally planned as a museum by
William Bullock, a Sheffield jeweller and
goldsmith who moved first to Liverpool and
then to London. He intended it to house his
personal collection of antiquities, weaponry
and natural history curiosities; all 15,000
exhibits which had taken him seventeen
years to accumulate. Accordingly, he called it
the London Museum and charged a shilling

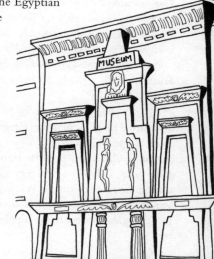

The Egyptian Hall – the Home of Mystery.

entrance or a guinea for an annual ticket. So successful was it that on the strength of the natural history exhibits he was elected a member of the prestigious Linnaean Society.

In 1816 he exhibited a series of Napoleonic relics, including Napoleon's carriage that had been captured at Waterloo. Almost a quarter of a million people paid to see the display, apparently generating him a profit of £35,000. Always an astute businessman, he clearly wondered whether he could better use the space and so three years later he sold the whole collection and converted the building from a museum into an exhibition hall. Then it became known as the Egyptian Hall.

The design of the building permitted it to be used for several exhibitions at a time. Benjamin Robert Hayden rented space in 1820 to show his gigantic painting *Christ's Triumphal Entry into Jerusalem*, which generated a handsome profit. Sad to relate, however, the artist fell into dispute with the Royal Academy and since he had accumulated considerable debt he committed suicide.

In 1821 the circus strongman, adventurer and collector of Egyptian antiquities Giovanni Battista Belzoni showed artefacts that he brought back from the tomb of Seti I.

The American showman Phineas T. Barnum (1810–91), who would become the first show business millionaire, later rented rooms to exhibit a series of spectacular 'freak shows' and to debut the appearance of General Tom Thumb.

In 1825 the bookseller and publisher George Lackington bought the Egyptian Hall and continued its tradition of exhibitions, albeit more artistic ones than the spectacular and bizarre displays of the showman Phineas Barnum.

THE MAGICIANS START TO APPEAR

In 1845 a stage act was booked at the Egyptian Hall. This was for The Mysterious Lady, an unknown veiled woman who would sit on a chair on the stage with her back to the audience, yet who could name the spots on dice or the numbers on cards when she had no possible way of seeing them. In addition, she could repeat snatches of conversation uttered in a whisper a considerable distance away.

A review in the *Illustrated London News* of 29 March 1845 expressed absolute amazement: '... [she has] a perfect knowledge of every circumstance that takes place behind her ...'

In 1857 the French conjuror Henri Robin appeared and presented a very full and varied magic repertoire. He performed sleight of hand, classic tricks, mental mysteries and illusions.

One of his most popular illusions, however, was called 'The Medium of Inkerman'. This was a reference to the Battle of Inkerman that had been fought during the recent Crimean War in 1854. A drum stood upon a tripod and eerily it would rap out answers to questions posed by the audience. Many left convinced that the answers were being supplied by a drummer boy casualty of the battle.

It was not just magicians who performed at the Egyptian Hall. Spiritualists performed there, too, since its ambience and air of mystery seemed so apt for public demonstrations of mediumship. And the people just kept rolling in.

JOHN NEVIL MASKELYNE

We need now to stop and talk a little about one of the most significant magicians of the Victorian era. In time the Egyptian Hall would become synonymous with him and it would become known as England's Home of Mystery. He is also very important because of his profound antipathy towards fraudulent mediums. As a magician he had the ability to see through their frauds and expose them.

John Nevil Maskelyne (1839–1917) was born in Cheltenham. He trained as a watchmaker and had a fascination with machinery all of his life. He also was an avid amateur magician and used his skill as a watchmaker to build mechanical toys and to invent various conjuring tricks.

The Exposure of the Davenport Brothers

It was because of his interest in magic that he was asked to join a committee of spectators to supervise a performance given by the Davenport brothers in the town hall. The task of this committee was to ensure that there was no trickery involved in their spiritualist demonstration.

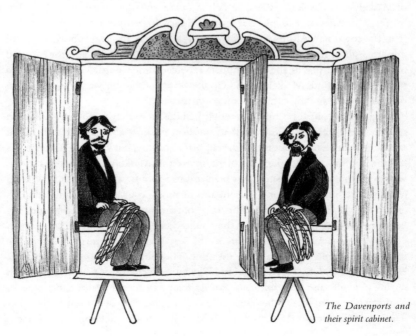

The Davenports and their spirit cabinet.

The date of the performance was 7 March 1865 and the hall was packed. The Davenports were on stage with their spirit cabinet. They entered the cabinet as usual and were duly tied up, hands and feet, and the knots inspected and scrutinised. Then the doors were shut and the curtains in the hall were drawn to exclude the afternoon light. Soon the psychic phenomena began. A tambourine was shaken, a guitar was strummed and a trombone made a noise. Then a door opened slightly, as it had done in hundreds of previous performances when instruments were tossed out of the cabinet, seemingly by spirit action. In this instance a curtain behind John Maskelyne stirred in the breeze and a shaft of light fell on the cabinet, allowing him to see inside. He saw Ira Davenport's hand, unfettered, about to throw a trumpet out. Fearing that he had been discovered, he dropped the instrument and pulled the door shut.

Immediately John Maskelyne called for the curtains to be opened and the cabinet to be examined. Inside the two brothers sat at either side of the cabinet just as they had been left, their bonds still securely tied.

Despite the remonstrations of Dr Ferguson, their front man, John Maskelyne strode to the front of the stage and announced that the performance had all been done by trickery and that he knew exactly how it was done. Further, he announced that within three months he would perform a show that would duplicate their effects.

On 19 June, together with a friend, George Alfred Cooke (1825–1905), who happened to be a cabinet-maker, the public saw the first professional performance of Maskelyne & Cooke. It was to be a close and (eventually) successful partnership for many decades. It took place at Jessop's Aviary Gardens in Cheltenham, rather than the town hall. Although they were not as slick as the Davenports they did duplicate all of the effects. The show was a resounding success and they gained much publicity, just as the Davenports received much negative press. On the strength of this both Maskelyne and Cooke gave up their jobs and prepared to go on a tour of the provinces as professional magicians.

They did, of course, become more polished the more they performed, although neither was especially good at self-promotion in those early days. Their initial success was dependent upon the Davenports exposure, but once the Davenports left the country to tour the Continent, interest in Maskelyne & Cooke's shows waned. Fortunately, their show was seen in Liverpool by an agent called William Morton. He offered to manage them and finance a tour, all they had to do was create the magic and perform. This they did and under his management they began to get major billings around the country and in London.

Their success was due not merely to the way that they performed, but to the scale of the magic tricks that they invented. They introduced a sensational 'Box Escape' in which John Nevil would be locked up in a chest that was encircled with chains and bells, and from which he would escape in an impossibly short time. In addition, they perfected a levitation illusion that looked totally impossible. *The Times* described it thus: 'The lady simply rises directly off the floor, where there is no trap, and remains suspended, full in the light, with nothing under her feet, over her head, or in any way visibly connected with her.'

But John Nevil's inventiveness went beyond that of magic. He devised several pieces of machinery and various mechanisms that were widely used. These included a typewriter, a cash register, ticket machines, telegraph apparatus and railway signalling devices. Between 1875 and 1913 he took out over forty patents on his various inventions. Most famously, he invented the locks that were used in public toilets for many years and which necessitated putting a penny in a slot to open the lock. It is from this that the expression to 'spend a penny' came from.

After appearances at the Crystal Palace in Sydenham and St James's Hall they rented a room at the Egyptian Hall in 1873. Their show was a sparkling success and they maintained their association with the Egyptian Hall for the next thirty years.

Psycho

The eighteenth-century magician Isaac Fawkes, known as Faux, used to exhibit an automaton in his performances. Such mechanical things had always fascinated John Nevil Maskelyne, for he had seen a mechanical bird in a cage, 'The Piping Bullfinch', at the Great Exhibition in 1851. It made a deep impression on him and he had been determined that he would build such wonders.

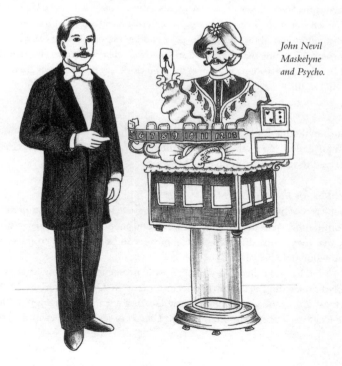

John Nevil Maskelyne and Psycho.

On 13 January 1875 he presented an automaton called 'Psycho' to the public. This was the small figure of a turbaned Hindu gentleman sitting cross-legged on a small box, which in turn was supported on a glass cylinder. Psycho was only 22in high, so there was no possibility of anyone being hidden inside. People were permitted to examine the doll itself, the box and the cylinder, to ensure that there was no machinery, no levers, pulleys or cords. They were then astonished when it was reassembled and it became animated enough to give the answers to arithmetic by selecting and indicating numbers, identifying cards or even playing whist. All who saw him were amazed.

Psycho is the figure of a small and melancholy Turk, with lacklustre eyes, and hands having a peculiarly unnatural appearance, even for an automaton, about the nails. He is seated cross-legged on a box, and he has small boxes near him. On the whole, he rather resembles a Turkish gentleman who, having determined upon travelling, had begun to pack up, and having suddenly tired of the occupation had sat down on a trunk, and rested his left arm on a couple of small boxes. However, Psycho is an independent gentleman, for he and his trunk are raised above the floor on a glass pedestal, quite transparent, and he most certainly appears to have no connection with anybody either on, or off, the stage. He does a sum in arithmetic; he takes a hand at whist, and plays (I was told this, not being a whist-player myself) a very fair game. Some clever people say there's a dwarf concealed inside. If so, the dwarf himself would be a fortune in a separate entertainment; but, again, if so, Heaven help that unfortunate dwarf! Where the poor creature can possibly conceal himself is, to my mind, a greater wonder than that Psycho should be worked by electricity, as was, I believe (for I dare not say I know) the plain clock face of transparent glass shown in MR. ROBIN'S entertainment.

Punch, *20 February 1875*

John Nevil added several other automata to the shows, including a mechanical woman called Zoe who could paint. None of them achieved the fame or managed to impress as much as did Psycho.

Witness for the Prosecution

For the rest of his life John Nevil Maskelyne stove to discredit fraudulent mediums, whom he felt were evil to prey on innocent people. He particularly disliked the way that they claimed to have special powers and simply used conjuring tricks to dupe vulnerable people.

In 1876 he was called as a witness for the prosecution at Bow Street Court in a Crown proceeding against the American medium 'Dr' Henry Slade. Dr Slade had been caught in the act of fraudulently creating a spirit message on a school slate. The case was reported in the *Illustrated London News* on 21 October 1876:

SPIRIT WRITING AT BOW STREET

The police magistrate, Mr Flowers, sitting at the Bow Street Court, has not yet concluded the preliminary investigation of the charge against 'Dr' Henry Slade. That noted 'medium' from America being a professor of the art and mystery of holding supernatural converse with the souls of the dead, has been accustomed to charge a fee of one sovereign for setting his deceased wife's bodiless spirit to write upon a slate. It is alleged by the prosecution that this is obtaining money on false pretences. The principal witnesses against Slade have been Professor Edwin Ray Lankester and Dr Horatio Donkin, who watched his actions while something was covertly written on a slate; and Mr Maskelyne the popular performer of conjuring tricks at the Egyptian Hall. The main question was, of course, whether the writing, which Slade exhibited to visitors as that of his deceased wife's spirit, was not in reality done by himself. The two scientific gentlemen had called at No 8, Upper Bedford-place, where Slade resided and exhibited. They found him there, with his assistant, Geoffrey Simmons, and having paid their money, they were treated to the spiritualistic performance. It appeared from their evidence that the slate was sometimes held by Slade with one hand under a table. This identical table was produced in court, amid much amusement. It appeared to be an ordinary kitchen table, with four legs and two flaps; its size when extended was about 4 ft square. It had the ordinary framework around the central portion of the table and the legs, to the depth of six or eight inches. When the flaps were extended it would appear to an ordinary sitter to be devoid of any framework. The table was turned over and examined underneath. It appeared that a single bracket, working on a pivot, opened out from the inner framework of the table for the support of both flaps.

Mr Maskelyne, when called as a witness, proceeded to direct special attention to the long movable bracket beneath the table, by which, he said, almost any slate could be supported. He suggested that the end of the bracket had been recessed to support the slate, but that this portion had been cut off before the table was brought to court. He never saw an ordinary table made in that way. He was next invited by Mr Lewis, the solicitor for the prosecution, to show the magistrate how the slate-writing might be done.

Mr Maskelyne, who was in the witness-box with a slate before him, said: 'It is a very good trick and the point is this. It seems impossible that a man with a heavy slate can hold it and produce writing with the same fingers beneath the slate. It is, however, very easy, especially if there is a slight projection or a peg beneath the table, or a cross-piece, as in the table in court, to push the slate against it and help to support it. The slate can then be supported by the thumb, and the whole of the fingers left at liberty. The best way, however, of holding the pencil – is not under a finger-nail, for that is impractical, but by an apparatus like this' – producing a little thimble, with attached pencil, fastened by elastic beneath his sleeve, which disappeared of itself when let go. With this instantaneously held on the end of his finger, he held the slate before him with his left hand, and, resting the thumb of the right hand on one side and having the fingers loose on the other side, he wrote a few words, which, when the slate was handed up to the bench, Mr Flowers read, amid great laughter, 'The spirits are present.'

Mr Maskelyne went on to say: 'The peculiarity of writing in this way is that the lines are necessarily somewhat curved. In producing such writing the operator would by a slight kick or shuddering take off attention for a second, and that would suffice for him to turn the slate over. Another short message would then be written on the under side, and on the slate being produced there would be the appearance of writing on the side which had apparently been next to the table. Having two messages written on a slate is, of course, convenient; for the performer would read the upper one and, rubbing it out, would say to his visitor, "You hold the corner." Of course, the point of the trick is that he turns the slate over, beneath the table, and then, after it has been held close against the table, the writing appears again.'

Slade was found guilty of obtaining money by false pretences and sentenced to three months' hard labour. But there was a technical problem and he was dismissed. Then, before further proceedings could be started, he and his assistant, Geoffrey Simmons, sailed for France.

Thus do the mighty fall. At one time Slade was said to be worth over $1 million, but thanks to an extravagant lifestyle and the disgrace that fell upon him after the exposure and subsequent legal case, his reputation was in tatters and he gradually drifted into obscurity and died a pauper.

Back in the United States a different version of his legal case was bandied about. It was said that he had been arrested and tried for fraud, but gained his freedom by allowing himself to be searched, handcuffed and blindfolded, then permitted to give a demonstration of his powers in the court. So impressive was his séance that he was immediately released with many apologies.

The Ghost of a Case

Not all of John Nevil's legal actions were so successful. One such case was an action that he took out against the Archdeacon Colley in 1905. Curiously, this had its origin in a case brought before the Huddersfield Magistrates Court in 1876, when a Dr Monck was accused under the Vagrancy Act of 1838. This would possibly never have come about had it not been for the Slade case that Maskelyne had been so involved in as a witness for the prosecution.

The Reverend Francis Ward Monck had been a clergyman at the Baptist chapel at Earl's Barton, but sometime in 1873 he became a devout spiritualist and began a career as a medium. He toured all over Britain and claimed to have healing ability. Accordingly, he acquired the title of doctor, despite having no medical qualifications. As noted earlier in the case of Henry Slade, this was not exceptional.

As we saw in Chapter 10 Materialisation and Chapter 11 Ghost Hunters and Psychic Investigation, Dr Monck acquired a significant reputation as a materialisation medium, and also as a slate-writing medium. In 1876, during a séance, a magician by the name of H.B. Lodge demanded that Dr Monck be searched. The medium took to his heels, locking himself in his upstairs room and then escaping through a window. However, incriminating evidence was found in the room, with dire consequences for him.

The Archdeacon Thomas Colley was a firm supporter of the medium, despite the evidence against him. In 1905, twenty-nine years after the case of Dr Monck, the archdeacon challenged Maskelyne and offered to pay him £1,000 if he could duplicate a feat of materialisation that he had seen Dr Monck perform. John Nevil duly did this, making a 'spirit' emanate from his side on a brightly lit stage. A critic of *The Times* wrote that Maskelyne had certainly won the challenge as a result. Nonetheless, Colley refused to pay, the result being that John Nevil sued him. The archdeacon countersued for libel.

This time John Nevil was unsuccessful, because Alfred Russel Wallace, another supporter of Dr Monck, and one who had witnessed the materialisation medium produce an ectoplasmic form, was called by the defence. A distinguished scientist, he said: 'I should call Mr. Maskelyne's performance an absurd travesty of what I saw and of what Archdeacon Colley describes.'

The court found against Maskelyne, who was made to pay damages and costs. Although it may have irritated him beyond measure to have lost the case, there was a spin-off. The publicity brought customers flocking to the Egyptian Hall.

The Latter Years

Maskelyne was a great magical inventor. One of the most famous of his illusions, which became almost a signature illusion of the Victorian magicians, was 'sawing a lady in half'.

His partnership with George Alfred Cooke came to an end in 1905 when George Alfred died. It was also to be the end of the Egyptian Hall, the Home of Mystery, for it had been gradually falling into disrepair. It was demolished that year. Yet it was not the end of John Nevil's career. Since 1893 a talented magician called David Devant had been performing there as well, by invitation of Maskelyne and Cooke. He had performed some amazing illusions, including 'Vice Versa', the transformation of a woman into a man, and the first stage version of the 'Indian Rope Trick'.

In 1905 they became partners and moved to St George's Hall in Langham Place. David Devant was to become the most significant conjuror of the early twentieth century and would become the first president of the Magic Circle when it was formed in 1905. He never used firearms, violence of any sort or abuse of animals. His approach was summed up in his catchphrase 'all done by kindness'.

But that is all quite another story of another century.

15

THE GREAT ILLUSIONISTS

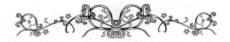

A Conjuror is not a juggler; he's an actor playing the part of a magician.

Jean-Eugène Robert-Houdin, the father of modern magic

The Victorian era saw many conjurors become stars of the fledgling entertainment industry. The size of their shows grew as their tricks developed from sleight of hand displays and tricks with small props to the grand illusions that demanded large stages. Many of the famous illusionists went on tour, crossing continents and building magnificent reputations as wonder workers wherever they went.

Although they were performing seeming feats of magic, they did not claim to have supernatural powers. They were quite frankly proud of their ability to honestly deceive. Those mediums who were engaged in fraudulent practices using conjuring techniques, on the other hand, were anything but honest. They were deliberately setting out to dupe people who were bereaved by conning them into thinking that they could actually summon up spirits and bring messages from their loved ones. This cold-hearted deceit alarmed and angered many magicians, such as John Nevil Maskelyne, whose conflict with and exposure of certain mediums we read about in the last chapter. Yet there were others who exposed deceit in its various forms.

THE WIZARD OF THE NORTH

The first of the conjurors who really made the switch from fairground entertainment to the stage, and elevated the position of the magician to that of national celebrity, was John Henry Anderson (1814–74). He was a man who understood the importance of self-advertisement and reputation building. His very title – the Wizard of the North – tells as much. The legend is that he was given the name by no less a national figure as Sir Walter Scott, after he had been entertained by Anderson. He had declared, allegedly, that whereas he (Sir Walter) was known as the Wizard of the North, it should really be a title used by Anderson. The story is fiction, for Anderson had not even started on his magic career before the great writer died. Yet of such stories legends are born.

The Wizard of the North was indeed one to foster legends. He claimed to have performed before King George IV (1762–1830) and King William IV (1765–1837). It is doubtful at the least to say that he performed before King George IV, since he had died before Anderson ever left Scotland for the first time. At the height of his fame his travelling shows were immense, necessitating several carriages, great trunks and always lots of advertising and street parades. It is said that his brashly coloured show-bills would go well before him and would end up plastered on the pyramids when he travelled to Egypt and on the cliffs of the Niagara Falls during his American tour. On his return from a European tour he had a huge poster designed, based somewhat on the famous painting *Napoleon's Return from Elba*. In it Anderson is depicted as a heroic figure surrounded by adoring spectators and with fanciful depictions of Nelson on his column doffing his hat to 'the Wonder of the World'.

His repertoire of tricks was vast, though not always of his own devising, and one was to become famous and would become the iconic trick of all magicians. This was the pulling of a rabbit from a top hat. Once again, whether he invented the trick or not, he took the credit. His other signature trick, catching a bullet fired at him, always came at the end of his shows to terrific applause.

John Henry Anderson was born the son of a tenant farmer in Aberdeenshire in 1814. He was orphaned early and entered the workforce at the tender age of 10 as an apprentice to a blacksmith, but he always had dreams of being first an actor and then an entertainer. When a troupe of touring players came to the area he was enchanted and left with them to make his fortune. It was while he was with them that he learned some conjuring tricks and began on the path that would take him around the world and lead to fame and several fortunes, which he would duly lose.

In 1837 he gave a magic performance at Brechin Castle to Lord Panmure, who wrote him a glowing endorsement: 'I have no hesitation in saying that you far excel any other necromancer that I have ever seen, either at home or abroad.' Anderson immediately used it on his advertising and found that vigorous self-promotion had a magic all of its own. People would flock to his shows.

Throughout his career he made and lost a vast amount of money. His theatrical persona was of a big man endowed with charisma and great politeness. In private he could be irascible and bucolic. He enjoyed strong drink and on occasions it landed him in trouble. In his career there were three fires that resulted in theatres being burned to the ground, one in Glasgow, one in America and one in London's Covent Garden, fortunately with no loss of life in any of them. His propensity to use methylated spirits and fireworks in his acts may have had something to do with this.

During his tours he taught conjuring to folk that wanted to learn simple card tricks and he also sold a 'Magic Dye' that would turn grey hair black in moments. There was, in other words, a dash of the mountebank in him.

On the other hand, he despised the new trend in spiritualism, for the Fox sisters had recently gained fame with their rapping séances. Anderson included a magic table that could rap out spirit messages in his performances, but without any serious claims of spirit involvement. He made no secret of his belief that they were simply using conjuring tricks.

In 1849 he gave a spectacular performance at Balmoral Castle before Queen Victoria. It was a great success. The young Prince Edward, who would become King Edward VII after the death of his mother over half a century later, was amazed, but said that his father, Prince Albert, knew how everything was done, of course.

In an extended American tour in 1860 he again did a trick that poked fun at the spiritualists. He performed a rapping trick in a theatre. It was in the run-up to the presidential election and the two candidates, Abraham Lincoln and Stephen Douglas, were busily campaigning. Someone asked Anderson if the spirits could name who would win the campaign. Anderson asked the ether if Lincoln was present and received a loud rap from the dress circle of the theatre. He then asked if Douglas was there and received another loud rap from somewhere in the stalls. He then asked who would win and seven loud raps rang out. It was assumed that this meant Lincoln, since there were seven letters in his name. Seemingly no one noticed that Douglas also consisted of seven letters. At any rate the exhibition of rapping was greeted with great applause.

It was a difficult time, however, for the Civil War was about to erupt, which it duly did in 1861. Despite this, Anderson had planned a tour of the south and sent his usual advertising bills in advance. It was not a shrewd move, for it was made clear that the Wizard of the North was not welcome, as indeed no one from the north was in those turbulent times.

His financial problems led him to keep touring his show right up until his death in Darlington in 1874. He was buried in the same plot as his mother in Aberdeenshire.

ROBERT-HOUDIN – THE FATHER OF MODERN MAGIC

A rival to Anderson was the French magician Jean-Eugène Robert-Houdin (1805–1871). In time he would eclipse him and earn the accolade 'the father of modern magic', gathering multiple honours and plaudits along the way.

He was born simply Jean-Eugène Robert, the son of Prosper Robert, a watchmaker in Blois. He took on the name Robert-Houdin when he married

Josèphe Cecile Houdin, the daughter of a Parisian clockmaker in 1830. It was a name that would go down in the annals of the conjuring art.

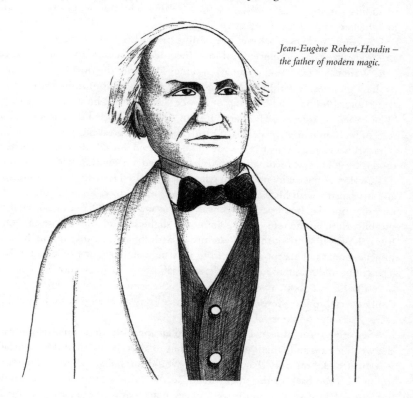

*Jean-Eugène Robert-Houdin –
the father of modern magic.*

As a boy, his father had ambitions for him and hoped that he would become a lawyer, so he was sent to the University of Orleans from whence he graduated at the age of 18. He was then apprenticed to a lawyer, but spent so much time making clockwork apparatuses and toys that he was sent home. This pleased Jean-Eugène no end for he simply wanted to be a watchmaker like his father. And so, he was apprenticed to his cousin.

It was in those early days that he discovered conjuring by accident. He had been waiting for some books on watchmaking to arrive at his local bookseller only to discover, upon getting them home, that they were about entertainment. They contained several conjuring tricks, which fascinated him. Apparently he stayed up all night reading them and even stole a street lamp because his own ran out of oil.

He joined an amateur acting group and started performing magic, eventually taking professional bookings. In 1830 he moved to Paris and there met and fell in love with Josèphe Cecile Houdin, with whom he had eight children. He went to work for her father, essentially spending his time inventing things in the workroom at the back of the shop. These included a whole series of automata, including singing birds. Sadly, only three of their children would survive and Josèphe herself died at the age of 32.

Jean-Eugène kept working and conjuring, in his spare time creating his amazing automata and mechanical toys. Included was a wondrous figure called 'The Writer', which could do amazing things like write the final lines of poems or draw pictures. It would be exhibited at the Paris Exhibition in 1844 before King Louis Philippe, the last king of France.[10] A year later he started to present 'The Fantastic Soirées of Robert-Houdin', which included his automata and feats of prestidigitation, or sleight of hand. They were a great hit.

Yet with a young family to take care of he still could not afford to go completely professional. He was fortunate then to have forged a friendship with the Count de l'Escalopier, a wealthy nobleman who much admired Jean-Eugène's conjuring and his artistry with his watchmaking and automata. Jean-Eugène confided to him that one day he hoped to become a great magician. The count offered to subsidise him, but he refused. The count felt slighted and left in a state of pique. It was, however, short-lived and he returned with the request that although Jean-Eugène would not accept a favour from him, he would beg one of Jean-Eugène. The count told him that he kept large sums of money in an escritoire,[11] but that over a period of about a year he had been systematically robbed. He had tried doing everything to prevent it, sending servants away, changing locks, putting secret fastenings on doors, all to no avail.

After some thought Jean-Eugène devised an apparatus that could be put into the writing desk and which would fire a shot to alert the house if the escritoire was disturbed. Not only that, but a claw would immediately tattoo the word 'robber' on the back of the thief's hand. To the count's great credit he would not use a device that would leave a permanent mark, so Jean-Eugène made adjustments so that the device would merely scratch the thief's hand.

The device worked and the culprit was found to be the count's 'faithful' retainer. The long and the short of it was that the money, 15,000 francs that had been stolen, was given to Jean-Eugène on condition that he use it to finance the special theatre that he had dreamed off, only paying it back when he could out of the profits from the theatre.

It was the start of a glittering career that took Robert-Houdin around the world. He invented illusions including a suspension trick that equalled anything that was done in the darkness of the spiritualists' séance parlours, and an illusion that depended on the newly discovered scientific principle of electromagnetism. This later illusion was called the 'Light and Heavy Chest', and consisted of a box containing a steel plate. When an electromagnet was switched on under the stage

10. Napoleon III would next rule France as the emperor.
11. Escritoire – a writing desk.

the chest could not be lifted, even by a strong man. He went on to improve it, even after the public became aware of the principle. Effectively he showed the magician's talent for misdirection.

Yet another that amazed audiences was his 'Orange Tree Illusion' in which an orange tree grew, blossomed and bore fruit as the audience watched. Oranges were plucked and tossed to members to show that they were genuine. Not only that, but a handkerchief that he had previously borrowed from a lady in the audience was found inside one of the oranges. Two mechanical butterflies then flew upwards carrying the handkerchief back to the lady.

He also devised a highly effective mentalism act with his son that he called 'Second Sight'. Again, it was as good as, or better than, the clairvoyant messages that many mediums purported to give.

One of the amazing stories about Robert-Houdin reads like a *Mandrake the Magician* adventure. He was sent by the French government as an ambassador to French-occupied Algeria because there was genuine concern that Algerian magicians were able to perform feats of magic which could incite people against the French government. These feats included eating glass and showing invulnerability to injury or to fire. His task was to demonstrate that his powers were superior to theirs.

Robert-Houdin used his magic shows to do so, including using the 'Light and Heavy Chest' with its electromagnetic secret. In addition, he had rigged it so that when one of the Algerian magicians touched it he received an electric shock which sent him scuttling from the stage.

He was a master magician who left a great legacy in the books he wrote. As we shall see later, he also influenced a small boy called Ehrich Weiss whose ambition it became to emulate him. The name he took was in honour of Robert-Houdin – thus Harry Houdini was born, the greatest escapologist of all time and one of the great scourges of fraudulent mediumship.

Robert-Houdin adopted an impartial attitude towards spiritualist mediums. One of the problems that he had was in being permitted to sit at a séance, since his reputation went before him. In his book *The Secrets of Stage Conjuring* he reveals the secrets of several major illusions and also devotes several chapters to the methods by which fraudulent mediums could easily produce their phenomena. In one chapter on spiritualistic manifestations he refers to the medium D.D. Home's levitations and then describes how this can be duplicated.

In another chapter he refers to the scientific method by which string instruments might be seen to play of their own accord. It was all based on the principle of resonance, which had been demonstrated by the physicist Charles Wheatstone (1802–75), an expert on acoustics, at the London Polytechnic Institution in 1855. He followed this up with his description of how to produce a rapping table. But most significantly, he gave a long description of the feats of the Davenport brothers and then followed it by a meticulous description of how virtually every part of their act could be duplicated.

HERRMANN THE GREAT

You will note that superlatives tended to follow the Victorian magicians. Many of them were perhaps not all that great, yet some truly were wonderful performers. Alexander Herrmann (1843–96) was born in France to German parents, but later in life, after a successful career in Europe and Russia, he immigrated to the United States where he continued to be a great success.

Magic was always in his blood and he worked as an assistant to his elder brother, Carl Herrmann. Carl was the eldest of the family of sixteen children and Alexander was the youngest. There was twenty-seven years between them so they never shared childhood experiences; the relationship being more like parent and child than siblings. Carl was already an established magician in his own right when Alexander was just a boy. He had performed in England and the United States, using a variety of titles, including the Premier Prestidigitateur in France and The First Professor of Magic in the World.

Eventually, after learning his trade, Alexander set off on his own and performed around Europe. In 1870 he came back to London to an extensive engagement at the Egyptian Hall. His appearance marked him out as a worker of wonders, for he was tall and slim, almost Mephistolean, with a neat goatee beard and always immaculately dressed in evening wear. He epitomised how a magician should look for most of the following century.

His illusions were big and spectacular and some were based on those of other magicians, such as Robert-Houdin. Nevertheless, he was also highly skilled at sleight of hand and extremely popular. Indeed, he gave several royal command performances.

One of his main assistants and stage manager was William Ellsworth Robinson, who would later find fame in the annals of medical history as the Chinese magician, Chung Ling Soo. His was a tragic story that we shall come to soon.

HARRY KELLAR

One of Herrmann the Great's main rivals was a magician who was often known simply as Kellar. He was actually born Heinrich Keller (1849–1922), but he changed the spelling and adopted the first name of Harry, since all his friends knew him thus. As a youngster he was apprenticed to a chemist, but after an inexplicable explosion occurred he decided to simply disappear rather than face the music.

Seeing a performance of a show by the 'Fakir of Ava', he applied for a job and was taken on as an assistant, where he gradually developed conjuring skills. Then he made an unsuccessful attempt to make it on his own as a professional conjuror. When the money started to get tight he obtained another job as an assistant. This time it was not to a conjuror, but to the spiritualistic demonstrators

William and Ira Davenport, whom we heard of in Chapter 14 The Egyptian Hall. It was not a happy period of employment, for the Davenports were secretive about their show and hard taskmasters. Apparently, after being publicly humiliated by them, Harry left, as did another assistant, William Fay. It was not a good turn of events for the Davenports, since Harry and William Fay set themselves up as a rival act, the difference being that they combined the cabinet trickery with lots more conjuring. They made no pretence of actually contacting the spirits.

The two conjurors separated eventually, each going their own way. Kellar became more and more famous and travelled with his show to London. There he saw Maskelyne and Cooke at the Egyptian Hall and, by all accounts, somehow acquired plans for some of the automata and illusions, which he reproduced in his own show. This included a version of the famous levitation illusion. Thus, it was not long before he was commanded to perform before Her Majesty Queen Victoria at Balmoral Castle.

While on a tour in India in 1882 he issued a challenge in the *Indian Daily News* to William Eglinton, the materialisation and slate-reading medium. Eglinton accepted and Kellar had to admit that some of the phenomena the medium produced seemed genuine. Upon slate reading, however, he reserved his opinion; there were certainly several ways that fakery could be achieved.

CHUNG LING SOO – THE MARVELOUS CHINESE CONJUROR

Chung Ling Soo was the stage name of the American magician William Ellsworth Robinson (1861–1918), who did his whole performance dressed as a Mandarin conjuror, without speaking a word. He famously died on the stage of the Wood Green Empire while performing the illusion of the 'Bullet Catch' between his teeth. He was accidentally shot and died the following day. There are several fascinating books about his life, including *The Riddle of Chung Ling Soo* by Will Dexter and *A Gift from the Gods: the story of Chung Ling Soo Marvelous Chinese Conjurer* by Val Andrews.

William Robinson was born in New York in 1861 and first surfaced as a conjuror in the 1880s as Robinson the Man of Mystery. Significantly, his act consisted of conjuring, mind reading and spiritualism feats. A good all-round performer, he played the variety theatres until 1887 when he met his wife, Olive Path, a petite lady who would work with him for the rest of his life.

With her he performed a 'Black Art' show. This he claimed as his invention. It consisted of a black backdrop which, with the stage lights directed slightly outwards towards the audience, allowed an assistant dressed entirely in black to be invisible. Thence all manner of illusions were possible – appearances, disappearances and levitations. He fronted the act as Achmed Ben Ali. In this he was demonstrating his love of acting and his fascination with the East.

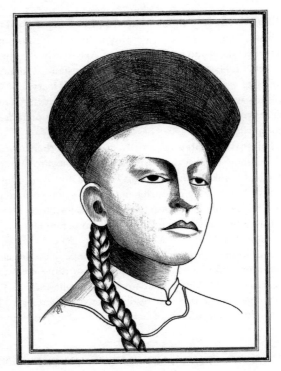

Chung Ling Soo – the Marvelous Chinese Conjuror.

His growing fame was such that he attracted the attention of the two big fish in magic, Herrmann the Great and Harry Kellar. Both offered him a job as their stage manager and assistant, but Kellar won. And so, as well as performing in his show, William was a backroom boy. This meant that part of his job was to invent tricks for the magician, rather like modern-day Jonathan Creek in the television series of the same name. It was an arrangement that benefited them both, but it was not so fortunate for many spiritualist mediums.

Kellar went about the country demonstrating just how phenomena could be produced. The black art method of Achmed Ali Ben came to its fore. Kellar had challenged a medium called Cary that he could duplicate his claims of producing spirits in a cabinet. Accordingly, he used the black art technique to 'produce' William and Olive.

In 1893 he left Kellar and went to work with Herrmann. There he learned a great deal about make-up and stagecraft from the older magician. He was, after all, regarded as the model magician. William was a natural at mimicry and disguise, to the extent that on occasions he understudied for Herrmann and no one was any the wiser – apart from when it was deliberately done with great flamboyance, such as the time that Herrmann had ostentatiously deported himself at a race meeting while William impersonated him on stage. News of Herrmann being able to be in two places at once enhanced his reputation.

William's disdain for spiritualistic trickery resulted in him writing *Spirit Slate Writing and Kindred Phenomena* in 1898. It is considered to be one of the classic books on the subject.

This thespian talent held him in good stead when he decided eventually to take on the persona of a Chinese conjuror. In fact, his reason for doing so was because of a financial dispute with another conjuror called Chung Ling Foo. This was a startlingly brilliant move which he carried off to perfection. He never spoke a word of English and was always attended by a small Chinese assistant, Suee Seen, who was none other than his wife, Olive.

Sadly, she was right beside him when one of the bullets that should have remained in its concealed chamber in the rifle was discharged and shot him. She was by his side when he died the following morning, bringing to an end the mystery surrounding one of the most colourful of the Victorian magicians, a scourge of the fraudulent mediums.

16

PEPPER'S GHOST

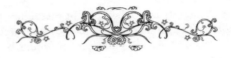

And then it started like a guilty thing
Upon a fearful summons.

Hamlet
William Shakespeare

In 1838, the year after Queen Victoria came to the throne, the very first polytechnic in Britain was opened in Regent Street in London's Westminster. It was called the Royal Polytechnic Institution and its original prospectus declared that it was 'an institution where the Public, at little expense, may acquire practical knowledge of the various arts and branches of science connected with manufacturers, mining operations and rural economy'. It exists to this day as the University of Westminster.

It was generally referred to as the Royal Institution, or even as just the London Institution, since it was unique to the capital. It was extremely popular among the general public for the public lectures and demonstrations that were given, especially since there were so many working models of the great Victorian inventions that were transforming life for millions of people. For example, people could take rides in a diving bell or see the newly developed science of photography in action.

In 1848, at the age of 27, a young man called John Henry Pepper (1821–1900) was appointed to the staff as an analytical chemist. He had a fine enquiring mind and a firm grasp of all of the sciences, yet, most importantly, he was an able administrator and an organiser of lectures, demonstrations and exhibitions. By 1860 he had become the director and was given the honorary title of professor. People flocked to his laboratory to see him demonstrate the latest scientific discoveries.

In 1862 Henry Dircks (1806–73), a retired civil engineer from Liverpool, visited Pepper and showed him a model of an invention that he had come up with to create a ghost on stage. He called it the 'Dircksian Phantasmagoria'. It did create an illusion, yet it would require a stage that was built with this purpose in mind. It would require a vast sheet of glass at the front of the stage and an open roof to the sky. The concept was terrific since an actor could be reflected in the glass to produce a transparent spectre. The problem was that it would only be seen at certain positions in the theatres and it was not practical. It was enough, however, to get the fertile mind of John Henry Pepper into action.

By Christmas he and Dircks came up with a much more refined method, whereby they could produce a ghost that would be seen by everyone in the theatre and which would not require a purpose-built theatre. Instead, the well below the stage would be used to conceal an actor. Immediately behind this a special slot was created so that a large glass sheet could be lowered by overhead wires until it was inclined at an angle of 45°. The stage lighting was arranged to shine outwards towards the audience rather than inwards onto the stage. Then, when the actor in the well was illuminated by a lamp, a reflection was seen in the glass, giving the appearance of a ghostly figure behind the glass. Another actor on the stage could interact with this phantasm, even apparently running it through with a sword. When the light was covered in the well, which of course was invisible from the auditorium, the ghost simply vanished.

Pepper demonstrated this effect to a small private group at the Royal Institution. Their collective reaction of astonishment was enough to make him see the possibilities that it offered. He and Dircks immediately patented their illusion. Then they went public.

PEPPER'S GHOST HITS THE STAGE

After a few small public demonstrations in which a skeleton dressed in a diaphanous robe was made to appear and haunt a poor student, before being stabbed and then vanishing, Pepper decided to use a proper stage. The performances became more sophisticated using proper actors and actual plays.

Charles Dickens' story *The Haunted Man* was performed, as was a scene from *Hamlet* wherein the ghost of Hamlet's father appeared in terrifying aspect. Unfortunately, the relationship between Pepper and Dircks became strained, basically because Dircks resented the acclaim that Pepper achieved. Although it was jointly their illusion and effect it became widely known as 'Pepper's Ghost'. And as an interesting optical illusion it is still referred to thus in physics textbooks.

The illusion was copied by many enterprising theatre owners, but was always quickly squashed when Pepper and Dircks sued. They held the patent and licence from them was needed by anyone else to perform the illusion. This led to a group of theatre impresarios attempting to break the monopoly by appealing against the patent. They claimed that there was no substance to a ghost and that there was, therefore, nothing to steal. After a hearing in his own home, the Lord Chancellor found in favour of Pepper and Dircks and the other side were faced with costs.

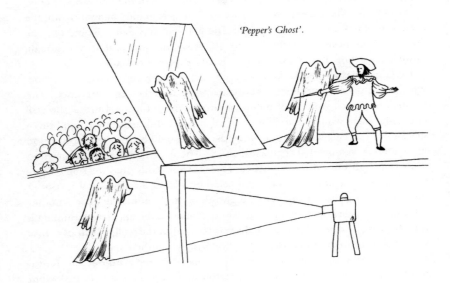

'Pepper's Ghost'.

The ghost shows were used by Pepper as a means of educating people about the use of optics, and also proved a considerable blow against the claims of spiritualist mediums who could not produce phantasms as convincing as 'Pepper's Ghost'.

METEMPSYCHOSIS – DONE BY MIRROR

The full 'Pepper's Ghost' illusion did require a large set and a lot of preparation. In 1878 Pepper also produced another optical illusion, together with an organ-builder called James Walker. He called this 'Metempsychosis'. In effect figures could materialise, dematerialise or be changed into other figures, or even into inanimate objects, literally before the eyes of the audience. No well was needed, just a small stage with three blue curtains.

It was done by having a large, specially prepared mirror fitted diagonally across the stage. It could be moved in a groove to produce the effects. One half of the mirror had the mirrored backing scraped entirely away so that it was simply plain glass. Then gradually the scraping became less thick, so that there was a gradual transition from glass to mirror effect. The mirror placed diagonally could not be seen, since it merely reflected the blue curtains. Yet a person, or whatever object was desired, could be secreted in the hidden triangular compartment behind. To make him, or it, appear the glass would be slid slowly so that the plain glass part would replace the mirror which was concealing him, and the effect would be a magical materialisation. To effect a disappearance, the glass would be advanced until the mirror concealed the person or object.

To perform a transformation the stage curtains at the front would hide an actor standing behind them, so that his or her reflection would make it seem that they were standing at the rear of the stage. If the glass was moved then the reflection would disappear as the mirrored part moved and the other actor or object would appear instead.

This effect was used in haunted house exhibitions at fairs and in the early days of cinema that were to follow, allowing for such transformations as man into werewolf or Dr Jekyll into Mr Hyde.

FINALE

Pepper and Dircks fell out and Dircks even wrote a book detailing how he had felt ousted by Pepper. Pepper himself fell out with the Royal Institution, with which his name had been synonymous for many years. He took his ghost show to the Egyptian Hall, but for some reason it failed to gather in the crowds. Indeed, he lost money on the venture and so, in an effort to recoup his losses, went on an international tour of the United States and Australia. Eventually, tiring of this curious science–cum–show business life, he went back to chemistry and settled in Australia for a few years, before returning to England. Once home he seemingly repaired his relationship with the Royal Institution and gave a few lectures on Australia before finally retiring.

When he died obituaries implied that his ghost had faded away before he had.

17

THE TRICKS OF THE TRADE

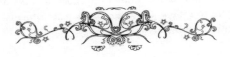

… they have at their command an army of beings unknown, indeed, but, in any case, of higher power than man; and by the aid of these supernatural powers, they actually – do what? Play the fiddle in a cupboard! Verily, demigods have become singularly unassuming in these days.

Opinion Nationale, 10 September 1865
Edmond About

The above extract is from the Paris press just two days before the Davenport brothers were due to give a performance of their travelling show. It illustrates that there was an air of antipathy towards their claims in some quarters. In no small measure this was due to news of John Nevil Maskelyne's exposure and his duplication of their show, as we recounted in Chapter 14 The Egyptian Hall.

Jean-Eugène Robert-Houdin, the celebrated illusionist, was eager to see their first show, but distance prevented him on this occasion, since he was busy performing in another part of the country. He was instead given a full account of what happened by a friend. In addition, he was able to read a detailed review of what was a calamitous debut in *Gazette des Etrangers* on 14 September 1865. The headline ran: 'Attack on the Davenport Brothers at the Salle Hertz.'

The article went on to describe a riot that broke out when one of the audience, an engineer, declared that the cabinet was rigged and that the whole thing was a hoax. The cabinet was damaged and the show ended after forty-five minutes when the hall had to be emptied by the police. Everyone was given their money back.

Robert-Houdin did see several of their shows later on and was of the view that they were simply jugglers employing conjuring tricks and had no actual communication with the spirit world. In his book *The Secrets of Stage Conjuring*, which was translated and edited by Professor Louis Hoffman,[12] he goes to great length to give a detailed description of the shows, and then systematically describes how they would have produced each effect.

Their show actually had two main parts. First was their 'public séance'. This involved their famous cabinet and was to be seen at relatively modest cost. The second part was a private 'dark séance' seen by only a selected few who had to pay an additional fee.

THE PUBLIC SÉANCE

This part of their performance was conducted with reasonable lighting, the whole mystery revolving around how the phenomena could be done in darkness within a cabinet.

The cabinet was separated from the audience by a railing about a yard high. It was a slightly made piece of furniture with three doors, the centre one having a diamond-shaped hole at the top. Inside there was room for three people to be seated or to stand. At either end were musical instruments, including a violin, guitar, trumpet, tambourine and bell. The cabinet was supported on two trestles, so that there was no way that any confederate could be hidden.

Before the start, spectators would be asked to inspect the interior and to stand in a circle around the cabinet, forming a ring by holding hands in order to prevent anyone getting near it to fabricate effects. The brothers entered the cabinet and were tied with their hands behind their backs and their legs tied to the benches. The two side doors were closed and no sooner than the middle one was closed, a hand of one of the brothers was seen waving through the cut-out section at head height. Moments later the doors were opened and they were both found to be free of their bonds. It was a remarkable escape, for the tying up had lasted ten minutes, the escape taking mere moments.

Then the cords were laid at their feet and the doors closed again. When they were re-opened the brothers were once more bound as before, the knots seemingly the same.

The doors were closed again and music started up – discordant noises from all of the instruments. An arm protruded through the hole and rang the bell. Then it and a trumpet were thrown out. Whenever the doors were opened the mediums were found still tied securely.

----

12. Professor Louis Hoffman (1839–1919) was a prolific writer of magic books. His book *Modern Magic*, published in 1876, is regarded as a cornerstone of conjuring. Harry Houdini described him as 'The brightest star in the Firmament of magical Literature'. In fact his real name was Angelo John Lewis, his pseudonym disguising his actual occupation as a barrister.

Next a spectator was invited to sit inside with them and he had one hand tied to one brother's knee and the other to the other brother's shoulder. Then when the doors were opened, he was found to have articles of the brother's clothing on him, while one brother was wearing his spectacles and the other had the spectator's cravat on.

Then, while they were still bound, flour was placed with a spoon into the hands of each of the mediums, the intention being to prevent them from making any move without getting flour on their clothing or scattered about the cabinet. The doors were closed and within moments they were opened to reveal that both brothers were free and yet they were still holding the flour in their hands. Both wore black suits and no trace of flour was seen.

THE DARK SÉANCE

The cabinet was removed and replaced by a small table on which were two guitars and a tambourine. The brothers would retire to another room to rest for a few moments then return and take seats opposite each other at the table. At their feet would be a coil of rope. The spectators, numbering fourteen or fifteen, would then be invited to sit around the table, each linking hands to form an impenetrable circle. The only lighting came from two gas burners at each end of the room. A spectator would stand by each and, on request, would turn them up or down.

At a signal from one of the brothers the room was plunged into darkness, and for two minutes everyone just focused on the stillness, listening for any noises. The lights then went up to reveal that both brothers were now tied to their chairs.

The lights went out again and the instruments began to play. Yet when the lights were turned up both of the mediums were still tied securely. Wax seals were made on the knots and the lights went out. Phosphorescent paint had been smeared on the guitars and tambourine. This time, as the lights went out, the instruments started to make noises and moved, floating into the air, hovering over sitters and ruffling their hair.

When the lights went on the mediums were still tied securely, the instruments just resting on the laps of sitters and the sealed knots still intact.

Then, to ensure that there could not possibly be any trickery, a sheet of paper was placed under the feet of each of the two brothers and a pencil outline of each was drawn around each boot. One spectator took off his coat and rested it on his lap. The lights went out again and the phenomena started. People were touched, hair was ruffled and the instruments were played. When the lights went up the mediums were still tied, but one was wearing the spectator's coat, while his own jacket was on someone else's lap. One brother was wearing someone else's spectacles; the other had another spectator's hat. Amazingly, the outlines were still there around their feet, showing that they couldn't have moved a muscle.

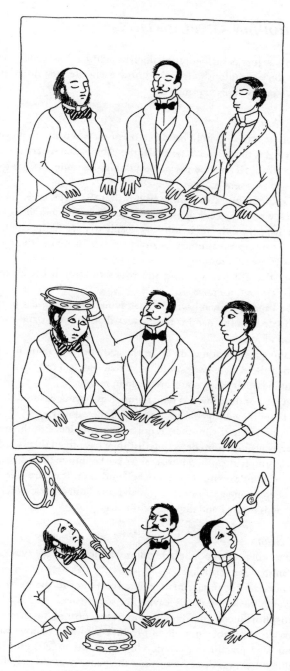

In the darkness of the séance a medium could play many tricks.

ROBERT-HOUDIN'S EXPLANATIONS

As the show was just described, the effects would have seemed amazing. But Robert-Houdin meticulously described how each effect could be performed. Here follows a précis of his explanation:

The Public Séance

The spectators are asked to hold hands – the reason is actually to prevent anyone from interfering. When they are seated in the cabinet the spectators are handed three ropes – this is to confuse the person doing the tying. He has to devise an impromptu way of doing it.

A trained escapologist knows how to position the body when being tied to allow for slack when he needs to escape – e.g., raising the shoulders, keeping the arms slightly away from the body, inhaling deeply to expand the chest.

Making a seeming involuntary cry of pain which makes the person tying subconsciously ease off pressure.

In making the escape, working the ropes to stretch the fibres, thereby lengthening it enough to move.

A trained escapologist will have practised lying the thumb flat in the hand so that when he does so the hand is no broader than the wrist and can be pulled through a coil of rope.

Most attempts at tying someone up by the audience will result in a slip knot.

The fact that there were two would mean that one had only to free himself in order to help the other. They could also help in retying.

Simple reversal of the moves to retie themselves, having ensured that they have secured the loops they escaped from on parts of the cabinet.

The spectator tied to the brothers is not an inconvenience to the mediums, but being tied prevents him from detecting that they have freed themselves.

The flour is simply deposited into a secret pocket inside their coats. They wipe their hands of the flour inside the pocket, and then they are free to do their manoeuvres before one gets a small bag with more flour from another pocket. He gives some to his brother and disposes of the bag.

The Dark Séance

So much of this depends upon it being done in the dark – the tying and untying all depend on the same principles.

Sealed knots do not in fact matter. The secret lies in the movement of the slipping through the loops, always leaving the seals intact.

The phosphorescent smudges are merely enough to show where the instruments are, but not enough to produce a glow to show anything that is happening. With practise one can develop the ability to see in the dark.

The outlined feet was done by turning the paper over after all the tricks had been done, then drawing an outline around each foot.

PROFESSOR HOFFMAN'S ADDITIONAL EXPLANATIONS

The additional notes by Professor Hoffman extrapolate from Robert-Houdin's masterly exposure and demonstrate how a medium can produce various phenomena at a small séance conducted in a private house. Again, a précis:

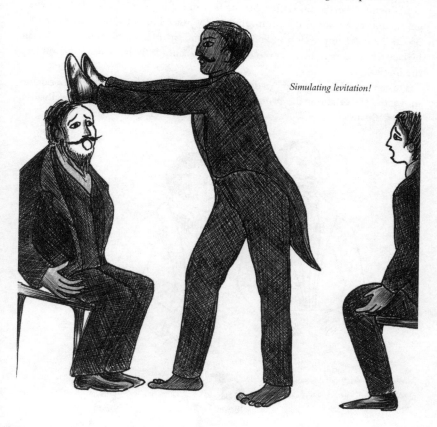

Simulating levitation!

The medium is placed between two people, who may be sceptics. If so they will be determined not to let go of the medium's hands. They are instructed how to hold the hands, by laying a little finger on the little finger of the person's hand next to them. The medium will probably inform them that if they go into trance, they should not pin their hand down, but should follow them. Thus a ring is formed at the start before the lights go out.

After a while the medium goes into trance and starts to have convulsive movements or twitches. He may shift his hands slightly and the people either side move their hands with him. One severe convulsive jerk results in a momentary freeing of the hand, which the sitter responds to immediately, placing his little finger on what he thinks to be the little finger of the medium's hand. Yet the medium has actually moved one hand entirely and has one hand touched by his two neighbours. He is free to make things move.

Another convulsive jerk and he can move the other hand. He is now free to perform more things; he can play instruments, blow a horn, shake a bell or a tambourine or make things levitate, or he can ruffle people's hair. He can even get up and move about the room. Indeed, by just telling people that he is rising he can give the impression of levitating up and up. Placing his slip-on shoes on his outstretched arms he can even touch people's heads with his 'feet' to complete the illusion.

He can operate a telescopic gadget, as small as a pencil, to make the tambourine move and hover about the room at a considerable distance, to give the illusion that it is floating.

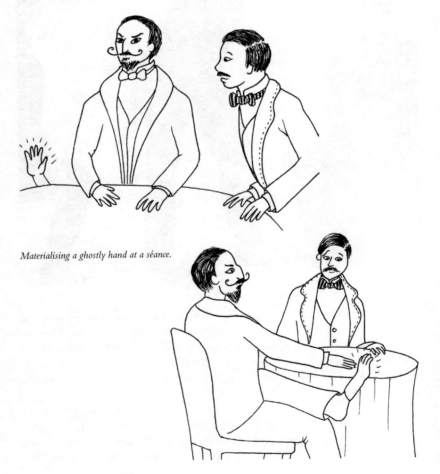

Materialising a ghostly hand at a séance.

And he can, if he wishes, make a spirit hand appear, merely by using a wax model. This is attached to elastic and secreted up a trouser leg. This is apparently an effect that Dr Monck used in his séances. He would use a square table and refuse to have anyone beside him. This would permit him to extract the dummy hand, slip it on a foot and, with it crossed over his knee, make it appear over the edge of the table. To make it disappear he would slip it off and the elastic would cause it to shoot back up his trouser leg.

All so simple, yet under the cover of darkness so effective.

18

THE KNIGHT, THE HANDCUFF KING AND THE ELECTRICAL WIZARD

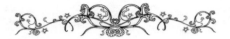

How often have I said to you that when you have eliminated the impossible, whatever remains, however improbable, must be the truth.

Sherlock Holmes in *The Sign of Four*
Sir Arthur Conan Doyle

We complete our journey with a consideration of three Victorian-born characters who really draw together the three strands of this book. The first is Sir Arthur Conan Doyle, an ardent supporter of spiritualism, spirit writing and spirit photography, who epitomised the Victorian Age of Credulity despite having created Sherlock Holmes, the most rational character in detective fiction. The second is Harry Houdini, the most famous escapologist of all time; a man who wanted to believe in spiritualism, but who was to become the greatest debunker of fraudulent mediumship. The third is Dr Walford Bodie, also a friend of Houdini, who was one of the most famous and controversial showmen of the Victorian era. He combined magic with exhibitions of healing using what he called his 'Bodic Force'.

SIR ARTHUR CONAN DOYLE

The creator of the world-famous consulting detective Sherlock Holmes is an enigma. On the one hand, he introduced the world to the Victorian underworld and created a detective whose deductive reasoning was nothing short of incredible. Holmes was a hard-nosed thinking machine who always sought a rational explanation for everything. On the other hand, despite all of his medical and scientific training, Conan Doyle himself was convinced about the existence of fairies (he was duped by several faked photograph of two young girls and fairies),[13] the truth of the spirit world and the ability of mediums to act as a channel between the two realms. His great intellect is in no doubt whatsoever, yet he was clearly a credulous man, a gift for fraudulent mediums. In a way he became the complete antithesis of Sherlock Holmes.

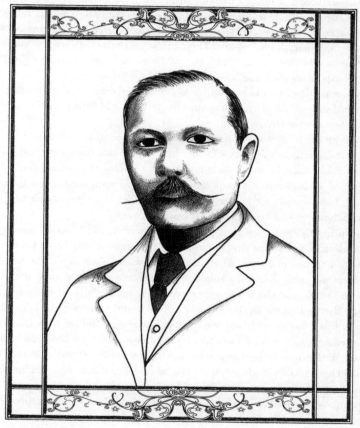

Sir Arthur Conan Doyle.

---

13. The Cottingley Fairies is the name given to a series of faked photographs taken by two young cousins, purporting to show them communicating with winged fairies. It was not until 1983 that the cousins admitted that they had faked the photographs with cut-out figures, although they maintained that they had actually seen real fairies.

Arthur Conan Doyle was born into a Catholic family in 1859 and was educated at Stoneyhurst, a public school in Lancashire that was run by Jesuits. It was a strict regime which suited Arthur very well and he excelled at sport. In later life he boxed and played cricket for the MCC, including one match in which he bowled out the famous Dr W.G. Grace. He played to a ten handicap at golf and he became the English Amateur Billiards champion. In addition, he was a balloonist, an early motorist, a pre-First World War aeronaut and a skier.

Medicine was his chosen career and he entered Edinburgh University, from whence he graduated in 1881. He worked as a ship's surgeon on a whaling expedition, before joining a practice in Plymouth and then setting up on his own in Portsmouth. It was there, while waiting for patients, when he started to write stories. In 1885 he completed his thesis for a doctorate in medicine on *Tabes Dorsalis*, a complication of syphilis. Then, in 1887, he wrote *A Study in Scarlet*, the first Sherlock Holmes novel, which was published in *Beeton's Christmas Annual*. It was the start of his glittering literary career.

He was sentimental and romantic and completely devoted to his mother. His father had suffered for many years with mental illness and Arthur had been forced to help support the family.

All of his life he had a strong sense of right and wrong and on more than one occasion came to the defence of those he thought had been wronged. In the famous Edalji Case, he successfully conducted a Holmesian investigation which vindicated an innocent man and went far towards inaugurating the Court of Appeal. In a second case he was responsible for securing the release of a man wrongfully imprisoned some eighteen years previously.

As a pamphleteer he was both prolific and effective, and a famous monogram of his played a significant part in reforming the divorce laws. Later, his writing advocating the use of the metal helmet in the First World War, and of the inflatable life jacket and collapsible India-rubber boats, undoubtedly saved many lives.

Since 1887 Conan Doyle had been interested in spiritualism. He maintained the interest throughout his life, but in 1915 a close friend of his wife had discovered that she had a facility with automatic writing, as indeed did his wife. This friend produced a message from Conan Doyle's brother-in-law, who had been killed in the war. Within this message were intimate details that Conan Doyle believed only he could have known about. It was the crucial evidence that he had searched for all of his life, and from then on nothing would convince him otherwise.

Spiritualism proved to be a great solace for him, for he had been depressed on and off for some years. He lost his first wife Louisa to tuberculosis in 1906, but married his second wife, Jean, the following year. Then the events of the war and its impact on his family hit him hard. His son, Kingsley, was wounded in Battle of the Somme and died of influenza during his convalescence in 1918. Then, within a few years, he lost two brothers-in-law and two nephews. Spiritualism gave him something to get his teeth into and he became a chief campaigner for the movement.

His book *The History of Spiritualism*, published in 1929, is an interesting history of spiritualism told from the inside. He is clearly supportive of several mediums, including Eusapia Palladino. In *The Land of Mist*, a Professor Challenger novel[14] published in 1926, Conan Doyle uses his masterly writing talent to take the reader on a journey into the world of séances and spiritualism.

Sir Arthur Conan Doyle died of a heart attack in 1930 in the hall of Windelsham, his house in East Sussex.

In the 1920s a curious friendship sprang up between Conan Doyle and Harry Houdini. It would not last because of the stance that they took at opposite ends of the spiritualist debate, yet both continued to respect the other and it is said that both regretted the rift that would come between them.

HARRY HOUDINI

Ehrich Weiss, the boy who would become famous as Harry Houdini the Handcuff King, was born in a Budapest ghetto in 1874. He was the fifth of seven children. His father was a rabbi who decided to immigrate to America to establish a better life for his family. At first they settled in Appleton, Wisconsin, then in the wonderful city of New York. Once there he set about educating his children and inculcated in all of them a thirst for knowledge and a healthy respect for books. He had high hopes of young Ehrich and wanted him to follow one of the professions. The last thing he thought he would become was a magician.

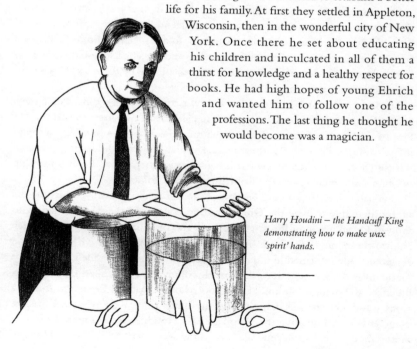

Harry Houdini – the Handcuff King demonstrating how to make wax 'spirit' hands.

14. Professor George Challenger was a character created by Sir Arthur Conan Doyle, who featured in five novels, including *The Lost World* and *The Land of Mist*.

Yet Ehrich was an avid reader and it was a book that converted him to the conjuring arts. As a teenager he bought a copy of Jean-Eugène Robert-Houdin's autobiography, *The Memoirs of Robert-Houdin, Ambassador, Author and Conjuror, Written by Himself*. Ehrich read it from cover to cover and decided that if Robert-Houdin could become a great performer with the world at his feet then so could he. From that moment on he practised conjuring incessantly. Cards, handkerchiefs and coins were easily obtainable and he built up his repertoire of sleight of hand tricks.

Rather like Conan Doyle, he had a deep respect and bond with his mother, and also like Conan Doyle he would lose his father relatively early and have to shoulder responsibility for the upkeep of the family. This was something that he continued to do throughout his life, gradually taking on responsibility for more and more people.

Also like Conan Doyle he was of an athletic disposition. Whereas Conan Doyle was a large man, Ehrich was small and lithe, yet he was fast and endowed with great stamina. He loved to exercise and made it a large part of his life. Indeed, in his chosen career his fitness, stamina and suppleness were key measures in his success.

He joined the Pastime Athletic Club and there he met Joe Rinn, who would also become a magician and stay a lifelong friend. It was he who first roused Ehrich's interest in spiritualism by taking him to a séance by Minnie Williams, a famous medium who lived on 46th Street. It is said that she had bought the house from a devout spiritualist believer who had been advised by the spirits to sell it for $1, not a cent more nor a cent less!

The séance was interesting to Ehrich. It was conducted in the light of a green lamp. Minnie had two hefty bodyguards in case any of the sitters caused trouble. From a spirit cabinet spirits appeared and moved across the room. Ehrich found it fascinating to hear the floorboards creak under their weight, having expected spirits to have no weight. At any rate he came away intrigued by the showmanship of Minnie, if not converted to spiritualism as a belief system.

Gradually, Ehrich started to get spots to perform his conjuring, which he did under the name of Eric the Great. Another friend of his, Jack Hayman, who showed Ehrich some of his first tricks, was also instrumental in helping Ehrich choose the name that would one day become synonymous with magic and escapology. He informed him that in French when an 'i' was added to a name it meant 'like'. Accordingly, since Robert-Houdin had for long been Ehrich's hero, he chose the name Houdini. He had not realised that the French illusionist's name was double-barrelled, having instead thought that Robert was a Christian name. Yet he did not like the sound of Eric Houdini, so considered that the most famous magician in America at the time was Harry Kellar. Harry Houdini certainly had a better ring to it …

In 1891 Harry Houdini decided that he was going to become a professional magician, so he gave up his job and devoted his energy to fulfilling his dream.

Significantly, it was about then that another book fell into his hands. This was *Revelations of a Spirit Medium, or Spiritualistic Mysteries Exposed – A Detailed Explanation of the Methods Used by Fraudulent Mediums, by A. Medium*. This book caused furore and was apparently quickly bought up and copies destroyed by frantic mediums. Harry was indifferent to spiritualism, but he saw the possibilities, and in the book he discovered all the various escape techniques used by such mediums to escape from their bonds in order to produce their phenomena.

Harry went on the road with his brother Dash. They toured in vaudeville as jobbing conjurors, the Houdini brothers. They were not hugely successful. Then, in 1893, he met Wilhelmina Beatrice Rahner, known as Bess, and they married. The result was that the act changed and Dash was replaced by Bess. From then on they were simply known as The Houdinis, and Bess would be his assistant for the rest of his life. They were devoted to one another.

Jobs were still not easy to come by and for a spell they worked in a medicine show called the California Concert Company, run by a 'Dr' Hill, who dispensed his patent medicine – Dr Hill's Elixir – throughout the show between the acts.

Dr Hill was a showman of the old school, never missing a trick or an opportunity. One such opportunity was spiritualism and he started promoting Harry as a medium. Harry duly introduced a mentalism and spiritualist component to his act.

This was not where his heart lay, however. He enjoyed the escapology part of his repertoire and saw the possibilities. Being the sort of man that he was he focused on that and gradually built up a reputation as the Handcuff King. He would issue challenges to the police departments in every city that he visited that he could escape from any set of handcuffs. And so he did. Then he increased the range of escapes, drawing more and more publicity as he did so. He escaped from cages, trunks, cells and even a milk churn. He did underwater escapes and aerial escapes from chains while hanging suspended from a crane, each stunt becoming more and more dangerous and more and more life-threatening. Some of these illusions became famous. The 'Milk Can Escape', the 'Overboard Box', the 'Chinese Water Torture Cell', to name but a few. In short, he became a star – *the* star. Then came movies and global celebrity. Later, he turned his attention to writing and wrote books that would become magical classics.

When his mother died in 1913 he was bereft. Although he had no real interest in spiritualism up until then, he desperately hoped that he would be able to find a medium who would be able to contact her spirit. While in England he had forged a friendship with Sir Arthur Conan Doyle, who was convinced in his own mind that Harry achieved his seemingly miraculous escapes by the supernatural power of dematerialisation. Harry could not dissuade him of this, nor was he swayed by Lady Conan Doyle's attempts to contact his mother's spirit by automatic writing. For one thing, she failed to appreciate that his mother had not been able to speak a single word of English. However, Sir Arthur's introduction to mediums was very useful to him. Harry took advantage of this and literally visited hundreds of séances, yet in none of them did he find anything other than tricks and platitudes. He made it his crusade from then on to debunk fraudulent mediums.

He did this by attending séances in disguise, together with a detective. At critical moments he would expose the medium, with drastic consequences seeing as though their acts were fraudulent.

In his book *A Magician Among the Spirits*, he recounted how the mediums perpetrated their frauds and he detailed how he had exposed Mina Crandon, a famous medium of the time. The book was a great success, but it effectively ended the friendship between Harry and Sir Arthur.

Harry died from peritonitis from a suspected ruptured appendix in 1926. It is likely that the appendix had been inflamed for several days, but Harry had refused medical treatment. The story is that a student struck him in the abdomen several times having asked him whether it was true that he could withstand a blow to his abdomen. Harry did not have time to tighten his abdominal muscles and received three blows which caused him to double up. Whether the blows had anything to do with the rupture of the inflamed organ is open to speculation. Nonetheless, Harry attempted to give a final performance that he was scheduled for at the Garrick Theatre in Detroit, but collapsed during the show and had to be revived. True performer that he was, he continued and finished the show, only then being admitted to hospital. He died a week later.

Yet that is not the end of the story. Before he passed away, he and Bess had secretly agreed that if one died they would attempt to send a message to the other at a séance. This message was something that only the two of them knew anything about. Sadly, although several mediums claimed to have made contact with Harry's spirit, the coded message never came through.

In an interview with Bess to the *Los Angeles Examiner* on 22 July 1935, she said: 'I receive many messages that are supposed to come from Houdini through mediums and strange séances but they never mean anything to me. Very often I go to séances, hoping and praying that the signals Houdini gave me will be heard. No message comes to me while I am waiting to hear.'

DR WALFORD BODIE – THE ELECTRICAL WIZARD

Our final character, Walford Bodie (1869–1939), was one of the most celebrated Victorian and Edwardian magicians. He had an act that used conjuring, hypnosis, clairvoyance and all manner of electrical gadgets. A self-aggrandiser par excellence, he styled himself as the British Edison, a nod at his inventiveness and his own regard for his genius. At other times he called himself the Electrical Wizard of the North in imitation of John Henry Anderson, the Wizard of the North, whom we met in Chapter 15 The Great Illusionists. Not only that, but he gave himself the title of doctor and added the letters MD after his name. As a result of the title and part of the act, it was widely believed that he actually was a doctor of medicine.

Walford Bodie was born in Aberdeen in 1869 and gained knowledge of electricity when he was an apprentice electrician to a telephone company. An interest in conjuring soon overcame any ambition to become an electrician, but the knowledge he gained gave him the idea to use electricity in his act. Dressed in an evening suit and sporting a huge upturned moustache, he cut a dashing figure as a magician. Indeed, the young Charlie Chaplin impersonated him so successfully that it gave him the start he needed in his career.

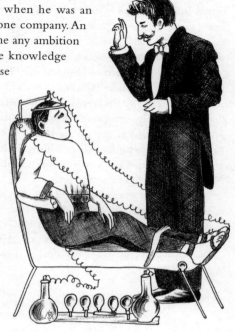

Bodie filled the stage with electric discharges and flashes. He passed 30,000 volts through himself and through volunteers. Hair would stand on end and he would illuminate sixteen incandescent bulbs and arc lights by holding them in his hands.

The centrepiece of his show was a mock electrocution, for which he built a replica of the

Dr Walford Bodie – the Electrical Wizard.

electric chair that was used in Sing Sing Prison in America. In this he would shock volunteers. In 1920 his friend Harry Houdini bought the original chair on his behalf and presented it to him.

Bodie also proclaimed his discovery of 'Bodic Force', which he claimed could be harnessed to heal people. He went further and established the Bodie Electric Drug Company, and used it to promote cures for the lame and the sick. Electric Life Pills and Electric Linament were eagerly purchased. He also used it to advertise his use of Bodic Force to perform bloodless surgery on people during his act.

In fact, Bodic Force was simply electrical stimulation and physical manipulation which he administered in a pseudo-surgical manner on people whom he hypnotised first. The power of suggestion, coupled with the demonstration of a seemingly scientific force that he had invented, would have been very strong. Many people received his treatment and many declared that he had cured them of all manner of ailments.

At the height of his fame he owned two hotels, a nightclub, a houseboat and a mansion in Macduff. In the 1890s he was the highest paid entertainer in the country and was earning a colossal £300 per night. His medical claims, however, outraged the medical profession and he was taken to task during one performance at the Glasgow Coliseum, where medical students pelted him with eggs and rotten fruit and fish. He had to beat a hasty retreat with cries of 'quack' ringing in his ears. Litigation followed and he was taken to task about his use of the title doctor and his claim to have an MD. He laughed it off, claiming that rather than standing for *Medicinae Doctoris* (Latin for doctor of medicine), his MD stood for 'Merry Devil' and 'Man of Distinction'. The publicity that he received did him little harm, for people still flocked to the music halls to see him perform.

Yet a new century beckoned and with it familiarity bred contempt. Electricity became relatively commonplace and his show lost its sparkle as, indeed, did he. His daughter died at the age of 18 and his son at 26. His wife of forty years, Princess Rubie, who had assisted him steadfastly throughout his career, died in 1931. He mourned her but soon found solace in the arms of his second wife, Florrie, a 22-year-old dancer.

Walford Bodie was an old stager. He kept performing until his death at the end of the season at the Blackpool Pleasure Beach.

A conjuror, pseudo-clairvoyant and 'healer', he could rightly claim to bridge all three areas of this book. The fact that his takings had diminished to a few pounds per performance is testimony that the curtain was coming down on the Victorian Age of Credulity.

SELECTED BIBLIOGRAPHY

PART ONE: MEDICAL MEDDLERS

Bartlett, E.G., *Healing Without Harm*, Elliot Right Way Books, 1985

Beveridge, A.W. & Renvoize, E.B., 'Electricity: A History of its use in the treatment of Mental Illness in Britain During the Second Half of the 19th Century', *British Journal of Psychiatry*, 1988 (153), pp. 157–162

Camp, J., *Magic, Myth and Medicine*, Priory Press, 1973

Darwin, C., *The Expression of the Emotions in Man and Animals*, John Murray, London, 1872

Drayton, H.S., *Brain And Mind Or Mental Science Considered In Accordance With The Principles Of Phrenology, And In Relation To Modern Physiology*, Fowler & Wells, New York, 1879

Dyson, L., *Doctor of Love – James Graham and his Celestial Bed*, Alma Books, 2008

Fowler, O.S., *Fowler's Practical Phrenology*, Fowler & Wells, 1853

Fowler, O.S. & Fowler, L.N., *New Illustrated Self-instructor in Phrenology and Physiology*, L.N. Fowler, London, 1870

Grierson, J., *Dr Wilson and his Malvern Hydro – Park View in the Water Cure Era*, Alpine Press, 1998

Holbrook, S.H., *The Golden Age of Quackery*, The Macmillan Company, 1959

Jamieson, E., *The Natural History of Quackery*, Michael Joseph, 1961

Lavater, J.C. (translated by Holcroft, T.), *Essays on Physiognomy*, Ward, Lock & Bowden, 1822

Lyons, A.S. & Petrucelli, R.J., *Medicine an Illustrated History*, Abradale Press, Harry N. Abrams, Inc., New York, 1987

Porter, R., *Quacks – Fakers & Charlatans in Medicine*, Tempus, 2003

Severn, J.M., *Popular Phrenology*, William Ruder & Son, London 1918

Sizer, N. & Drayton, H.S., *Heads and Faces and How to Study Them*, Fowler & Wells, New York, 1885

Souter, K., *Cure Craft — traditional folk remedies and treatment from antiquity to the present day*, C.W. Daniel Company, 1995

———, *Doctors' Latin*, Robert Hale, 2006

Vago, A.L., *Orthodox Phrenology*, Vago, 1875

Waxman, D., *Hartland's Medical & Dental Hypnosis*, Bailliere Tindall, 1989

Wells, S.R., *How to Read Character*, Samuel R. Wells, New York, 1870

Wynbrandt, J., *The Excruciating History of Dentistry — toothsome tales & oral oddities from Babylon to Braces*, St Martin's Griffin, New York, 1998

PART TWO: MEDIUMS

Bessey, M., *A Pictorial History of Magic and the Supernatural*, 1961

Crowe, C., *The Night Side of Nature, or Ghosts and Ghost-seers*, Aquarian Press, 1986 (reprinted)

Doyle, A.C., *History of Spiritualism*, the Echo Library, 2007 (originally published 1926)

———, The Land of Mist, in the Complete Professor Challenger Stories, John Murray, 1963 (reprint)

London Dialectical Society, *Report on Spiritualism of the Committee of the London Dialectical Society together with the evidence, oral and written and a selection of the correspondence*, London, 1873

Pearsall, R., *The Table-Rappers — The Victorians and the Occult*, Sutton Publishing, 2004

Spence, L., *An Encyclopedia of Occultism*, Dover 2003 (originally published Routledge, 1920)

Wallace, A.R., *On Miracles and Modern Spiritualism*, London, 1875

Wilson, C., *Psychic Detectives — the story of Psychometry and Paranormal Crime Detection*, Pan, 1984

PART THREE: MAGICIANS

Andrews, V., *A Gift from the Gods: the story of Chung Ling Soo Marvelous Chinese Conjurer*, Goodliffe, 1981

Bailey, M., *The Magic Circle — Performing Magic through the Ages*, Tempus, 2007

Budge, E.A.W., *Egyptian Magic*, K. Paul, Trench, Trubner, London, 1899

Christopher, M. & Christopher M., *The Illustrated History of Magic*, Carroll & Graf, New York, 2006

Clafin, E. & Sheridan, J., *Street Magic — an Illustrated History of Wandering Magicians and their Conjuring Arts*, Dolphin Books, New York, 1977

Dexter, W., *The Riddle of Chung Ling Soo*, Arco, New York, 1955

Gresham, W.L., *Houdini: The Man Who Walked Through Walls*, Holt, Rhnehart and Winston, 1959

Hopkins, A.A., *Magic: Stage Illusions, Special Effects and Trick Photography*. Munn & Co, New York, 1898

Houdini, H., *A Magician Among the Spirits*, (new edition) Cambridge university Press, 2011

————, *Miracle Mongers and their Methods*, E.P Dutton & Co, 1920

Lamb, G., *Victorian Magic*, Routledge & Kegan Paul, London, 1976

Lamont, P., *The Rise of the Indian Rope Trick – the biography of a legend*, Little, Brown, 2004

Robert-Houdin, J.E., *The Secrets of Stage Conjuring*, George Routledge & Son, 1900

Steinmyer, J., *Art & artifice and Other Essays on Illusion*, Carroll & Graf, 2006

Waters, T.A., *Encyclopedia of Magic and Magicians*, Facts on File publications, 1988

GENERAL

Dickens Jnr, C., *Dickens's Dictionary of London 1888*, Old House Books, 2006 (reprinted)

Jackson, L., *A Dictionary of Victorian London – An A–Z of the Great Metropolis*, Anthem Press, 2006

INDEX

Other titles published by The History Press

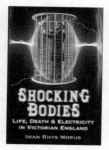

Shocking Bodies: Life, Death and Electricity in Victorian England
IWAN RHYS MORUS   £12.99

Here Morus explores how the Victorians thought about electricity, and how they tried to use its intimate and corporeal force. This is the story of how electricity emerged as a powerful new tool for making sense of our bodies and the world around us.

978-0-7524-5800-7

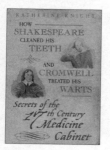

How Shakespeare Cleaned his Teeth and Cromwell Treated his Warts
KATHERINE KNIGHT   £12.99

A fascinating romp through seventeenth-century medicine and cosmetics. Documenting the all-important use of household substances and do-it-yourself remedies, this book looks at the emergence of modern medicine from everyday cures such as herbs, oils and foods.

978-0-7524-4027-9

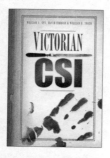

Victorian CSI
WILLIAM GUY, DAVID FERRIER & WILLIAM SMITH   £12.99

These selections derive from the final edition of Guy's *Principles of Forensic Medicine*. With original woodcuts, case studies and notes on identifying the corpse and walking the crime scene, Victorian CSI will fascinate lovers of crime fiction and of true crime alike.

978-0-7524-5513-6

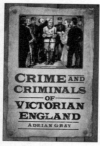

Crime & Criminals of Victorian England
ADRIAN GRAY   £14.99

This thrilling book not only recounts the classic Victorian murders, but also uncovers the wicked, the vengeful, the foolish and the hopeless amongst the criminal world of the time. You will encounter women who sold their children, corrupt bankers, the first terrorists, bloodthirsty mutineers and petty thieves; you will meet the 'mesmerists' who fooled a credulous public, and even the Salvation Army band that went to gaol.

978-0-7524-5280-7

Visit our website and discover thousands of other History Press books.

www.thehistorypress.co.uk